The Velocity
of Information

The Velocity of Information

Human Thinking During Chaotic Times

David P. Perrodin

ROWMAN & LITTLEFIELD

Lanham • Boulder • New York • London

Published by Rowman & Littlefield
An imprint of The Rowman & Littlefield Publishing Group, Inc.
4501 Forbes Boulevard, Suite 200, Lanham, Maryland 20706
www.rowman.com

86-90 Paul Street, London EC2A 4NE, United Kingdom

British Library Cataloguing in Publication Information Available

Library of Congress Cataloging-in-Publication Data

Names: Perrodin, David P., 1971- author.
Title: The velocity of information : human thinking during chaotic times / David P. Perrodin.
Description: Lanham : Rowman & Littlefield, [2022] | Includes bibliographical references and index. | Summary: "This book will appeal to a general adult audience interested in contemporary scholarly work about human behavior, chaos, and history"—Provided by publisher.
Identifiers: LCCN 2021055273 (print) | LCCN 2021055274 (ebook) | ISBN 9781475865448 (cloth) | ISBN 9781475865455 (paperback) | ISBN 9781475865462 (epub)
Subjects: LCSH: Human information processing | Thought and thinking. | Human behavior.
Classification: LCC BF444 .P478 2022 (print) | LCC BF444 (ebook) | DDC 153—dc23/eng/20220106
LC record available at https://lccn.loc.gov/2021055273
LC ebook record available at https://lccn.loc.gov/2021055274

∞ ™ The paper used in this publication meets the minimum requirements of American National Standard for Information Sciences—Permanence of Paper for Printed Library Materials, ANSI/NISO Z39.48-1992.

Contents

Preface

Chaos events, and the human reaction to them, have been a particular focus of interest for me throughout my career as an expert in school and community safety. Watching events develop and unravel in real time through the inception and duration of the COVID-19 pandemic prompted me to do a more formal analysis of individual and population-level behaviors in uncertain times.

This once-in-a-hundred-years' pandemic gave me firsthand experience; I was an active participant in field study, not merely an observer or spectator. I was embedded (alongside you, the reader) and immersed into society that was experiencing the COVID-19 pandemic, gaining real-world, real-time comprehension into how people see and react to a world plunged into chaos. Data and insight rich, I conducted a comparison analysis of current chaos to other chaotic periods in history.

This book rigorously clarifies and deepens how we think about a significantly uncharted area explaining societal human behavior during days, weeks, months, or even years of chaos. It delivers an indispensable scholarly review and understanding to population-level chaos events.

Here, I provide you with an expectation of how both individuals and the masses will behave during different stages of chaos. By anticipating those behaviors, individuals can position themselves out of harm's way and also ahead of the pack. This book provides a counterweight to the gravity of entropy that people and systems endure during prolonged uncertain times.

I explore the effect of time perception during traumatic events and the human ability to discern factual information through observation of seemingly mundane details. Psychologically, humans have cognitive limitations when faced with emergency events, and this effect is compounded by age and when there is uncertainty as to when the crisis will end.

There are a host of compelling and sometimes reclusive or difficult-to-access characters in this book, many of whom I have personally interviewed, who provide their recollections and hindsight advice for surviving chaotic times. Interestingly, people tend to react similarly when faced with uncertain and dangerous conditions.

The rate at which we process available information and how we choose to respond to different types of chaos are all dependent on . . . *The Velocity of Information.*

David P. Perrodin, Ph.D.

Acknowledgments
Member Checks

I would like to express my gratitude to the following individuals whose support and insight were invaluable in the development of this book.

Kerrie Ackerson
Drew Baye
Bryan M. Bowden
Juan Browne
James David Dickson
Joe Dolio
Glynn Foxx
Philipp Heinrich
Larry Lawton
Charles Mak
Clay Martin
Dr. David Mays
Dr. Paul Rapp
Nikolai Razouvaev
Morgan Rogue
Aaron Sawyer
Linda Stone
Robert Travis

I am also indebted to Aimee K. DiStefano for interpreting and evolving my doodles into the compelling graphics contained in this book.

Introduction

The early twenty-first century is a time when "information," like low-cost food is readily available almost everywhere in the West. With the proliferation of smartphones and public Wi-Fi, most of us carry devices that enable us to reach and be reached by any number of databases, media outlets, and individual content creators of varying quality and intent.

The same technology that allows us to connect with people we know and trust all over the world keeps us awash in nonstop waves of others' narratives, data, and arguments designed to change our minds and, subsequently, our behavior. "Electric circuitry has overthrown the regime of 'time' and 'space' and pours upon us instantly and continuously the concerns of all other men."[1]

In this unprecedented time when anyone with a cell phone can become a paid, professional "journalist," and when corporate media, in varying degrees, employ techniques and standards of citizen journalism, how does the individual make sense of all of this information raining down from the "cloud?"

Most of us have no problem distinguishing between the fast-food drive-thru and the fresh vegetable aisle at the grocery store with respect to the nutrient quality of our food choices. However, how does one distinguish between junk content and quality information? Currently, our information is all presented in much the same format and production value, and produced and edited to appeal to the specific biases and agendas of an individual's or company's target demographics.

How does the general population make sense of it all and learn to distinguish between and evaluate waves of facts, opinions, and sources without wearily or skeptically rejecting everything on the one hand or becoming too easily manipulated on the other?

These are not simple questions with simple answers, nor can the approach be a simple one. It would be easy simply to attack "the media" as a monolithic boogeyman attempting to deceive the public and push them in specific directions on behalf of establishment benefactors, but that is not the purpose of this book. The purpose of this book is to examine the challenges involved in obtaining valid information to supply our decision-making when faced with challenges and crises.

This issue is not merely a technological problem. Human psychology—our beliefs, fears, and biases—determines how we process the flood of information at our disposal, as well as how we are affected by it. Our challenge then is as psychological as it is technological; it is emotional as much as informational.

The trouble with humans is that our ability to process information is often influenced by our instinctive tendency to pursue pleasure and avoid pain. As far back as the seventeenth century, philosopher and physician John Locke considered the influence of pleasure and pain on knowledge derived through sense experience in his 1689 seminal work on epistemology, *An Essay Concerning Human Understanding*.[2]

In the essay, Locke argues that learning and thinking are distorted or prevented when juxtaposed with physical or mental pain.[3] When we are suffering, our minds are focused on eliminating the suffering, not on thinking clearly about its causes or effects.

Most people unaccustomed to dealing with severe and sudden changes to their comfortable and comforting routines seek to avoid or eliminate the uncomfortable chaos and confusion in which they find themselves.

This quandary presents a twofold challenge: that of dealing with the immediate—and, perhaps, ongoing—emotional pain of an extreme situation we are not prepared for while still needing to identify and process necessary information for navigating the hours, days, or months ahead.

This book presents approaches for dealing with this twofold challenge by analyzing crisis events in recent history and learning what they can teach us about how such intrusions of chaos into our daily lives affect our ability to gather and process the information we need to function in dynamic situations.

We will also share the firsthand accounts and reactions of individuals from around the world who have found themselves suddenly and unexpectedly facing such events. These recollections and analyses provide the reader with heuristics, or problem-solving strategies, for successfully dealing with chaos at the speed of information in their own lives. This book is practical advice for the next emergency.

EVALUATING CHAOS EVENTS

During any crisis, there are more questions than answers. Questions arise, especially in the early hours of each chaotic event, when alerts screech on our cell phones and torrents of conflicting, yet urgent messages gush from media outlets. What is the magnitude of the crisis? What is the cause of it, and what action should people take to protect themselves?

The speed of these details is known as the *velocity of information (VOI)*. The VOI can overwhelm and distress people who have not built a network of trustworthy sources and who do not understand the psychology of chaos.

Our inability to juggle multiple facts and opinions during chaos events drives us to plunge frantically into the datastream of TV, social media, and contacting friends and family to retrieve evidence that supports our beliefs. We then cobble together, conflate, and convincingly pronounce our findings to family, friends, and strangers on the Internet who have harvested information from the same headlines we skimmed five minutes ago.

Human beings seek confirmation bias. We want assurance that things will *return to normal* because we expend less energy to spin around a known torus than to plot a course in unfamiliar surroundings. We also want our beliefs to be validated and will therefore yield preference to what we want to hear over what we need to hear.

By tapping into external sources, such as twenty-four-hour news streamed to our phones, we dismiss what should be corroborated by observing what is happening directly in front of our faces. How often do you say, "I observed?"

Worse yet, even when we are indirectly affected by the crisis, we may personalize the event through media exposure or see ourselves as potential victims and inject skewed perceptions into already cloudy narratives.

Stop outsourcing your thinking. The more you steer your own wheel, the harder it becomes for others to steer you.

OVERARCHING CONCEPTS AND THE SEVEN PARTS OF THIS BOOK

In order to understand which information has real value, there are a few terms we can use. *Face validity* is whether something observed measures what it claims to measure, and what we are observing. A thermometer reporting 80 degrees Fahrenheit during a snowstorm would not pass face validity. It is either broken or your senses are deceiving you.

Member checks, or mustering a network of reliable confidantes across the country (or globe) to tell you what they are observing and experiencing with their senses in their local settings, can back up face validity. Using member checks helps to ensure that details come from an array of credible sources. What are your member checks observing? Does it match what you are observing?

You may have observed that toilet paper and pasta are among the first items that panicked people wipe from store shelves. However, when paint and puzzles sell out, the nuanced observer recognizes a crossed threshold into what is known as *"crowd-in" psychology*; essentially, when people feel the need to surround themselves with "comfort" items because they expect it will be months or years before their lives return to normal.

How do you interact with people who are bracing for extended disruption of their lives? How does information change during a prolonged crisis such as the 1986 Chernobyl nuclear power plant fire or the COVID-19 pandemic? How does the VOI change?

Observations of civilian morale during times of extended strife caused by economic depressions, natural disasters, and military conflict suggest that people in those perpetual stress environments began to lose hope after ninety days, leading to a cascade of adverse effects from depression to violence.

And for combat soldiers in months-long tours, complete psychiatric collapse was inevitable. World War II military field psychiatrist Dr. John Appel made note of the phenomenon of *finite voltage*. Every soldier not wounded or killed would sooner or later break down. What could be done to alter that statistical certainty?

It is well-documented that, during wartime, government public propaganda units put a fresh spin on the situation roughly every few months. That strategy included naming something a "new phase" or promoting a unifying event such as the scrap metal drives of World War II.

During the 2020 COVID-19 lockdowns, city parades for medical staff and (some) essential workers disrupted the "stay-at-home" languishing, framed the condition as transitory, and served to boost civilian morale.

Understanding how to navigate the VOI will help people survive prolonged chaos events by teaching the value of using face validity and member checking to make decisions based on trustworthy information. These are valuable skills during times of crisis as well as during everyday life.

For readability, this book is broken into seven parts. Part 1 of the book describes routines and the pace of information on typical days. We will refer to this as the "torus" and represent it as an inner tube. You may recall that in *School of Errors*, we referred to the torus as one's "bagel."[4] The bagel was a metaphor for our personal world as our minds see it.

Our daily lives traverse in a circle (days) and within the bagel's crusty edges (typical experiences across a small range or "normal"). Torus is our comfort zone. And not to snatch away your delicious bagel, but for this book, we will represent our torus as an inner tube.

We begin our day afloat on our tube and then slowly rotate through our day until we make it back to the start twenty-four hours later. Your torus is your typical day. However, life is unpredictable. What you know or think you can expect may change in an instant. Sometimes that may seem like bumping over rapids in your inner tube and simply having to grip tighter to maintain your torus; other times, it may seem like being unexpectedly flipped off your torus entirely, head underwater, not knowing what is happening.

The pace of your routines can be violently disrupted. Information from many sources is hastily blasted at you and can quickly become overwhelming. You are off your torus and in the water. Did something just brush my foot? How deep is this water? Someone laughs, someone else yells, *Shark!*

In our society and our media, being first and gaining attention is often valued over being right. In our technology-driven world, when we seek information, the algorithms and databases fire up quickly. Information is matched to our unique profile, and a powerful, bruising firehose of relentless data incapacitates us.

It is this particular equation of the speed and direction of information (velocity) that we will examine to give us the best clues for how to identify trustworthy information critical to our survival in all types of weather.

Linda Stone is a writer, speaker, and consultant who had spent the majority of her early career in executive positions at Microsoft tackling research regarding virtual (online) communities. Linda Stone's work informs us that we use our attention rapidly and serially. *Continuous partial attention* sets a cornerstone for later investigations of the links between attention and civilian morale during uncertain times.

We will deconstruct time into psychological time and physical time. We will understand how the phenomenon of *time dilation* during prolonged chaos events negatively impacts groups of people, especially children, while having nearly opposite—even liberating—effects on others.

We will learn how to recognize *indicators* and also examine how we use *heuristics*, which are essentially mental shortcuts that allow us to solve problems and make judgments quickly and efficiently, without constantly stopping to think about our next course of action.

We will discuss how using heuristics helps us become adept at storing information in the environment through a process that is called *cognitive offloading*. More importantly, we will show how these shortcuts can short circuit during chaos events.

Part 2 introduces us to former Soviet cyclist Nikolai Razouvaev and his experience acquiring information about the unfolding Chernobyl nuclear reactor accident—all as he prepared to race in nearby Kiev. While cycling past hundreds of lead-covered evacuation buses, Nikolai gained firsthand information that did not match the state media's official narrative.

He cautiously navigated Russia's secretive culture to acquire life-saving intelligence. His use of face validity was enhanced by a reliable member check network of people sharing authentic encounters with their surroundings and placing them against reports provided by Soviet party leaders.

Part 3 demonstrates broadening face validity by teaching you how to build a carefully vetted, trained, and coached group of analytical thinkers who are able to observe authentically and report what they experience in their environments. Through analysis of information production, you will be able to convert basic information from all sources into actionable intelligence.

Part 4 describes the behavior of soldiers and civilians months into a continuous chaos event. During the Second World War, U.S. Army field psychiatrist Dr. John Appel studied soldiers fighting on the front lines and determined a finite day count by which they would be killed, captured, or suffer a mental collapse. Observations of civilian populations reveal a similar finite voltage threshold. We will shed light on the characteristics of people approaching finite voltage and look into strategies to build individual and group resilience.

Part 5 of the book returns to human psychology and the infrequently observed phenomenon of crowd-in behavior that happens months into a chaotic event. Crowd-in behavior is easy to observe in consumer habits and also signals that people expect a chaos event to continue for months or years.

Last observed on a world level in the 1930s economic depression, crowd-in behavior returned in the spring of 2020. Did you notice that December's holiday decorations stayed up well into March?

Part 6 explains chaos and the subtle or sudden events that bring it into our lives. Unlike other works that portray chaos as binary (either present or not), this book introduces distinct markers denoting stages of chaos and shows that chaos occurs on a continuum impacted by time and intensity.

A "no-way-out" racing wildfire in the Smoky Mountains presents differently on the continuum than tracking the changing hours of operation at the local grocery store three months into a pandemic. We will define the characteristics of the four stages of chaos and examine the features of chaos events that last for months or years.

Part 7 examines the collective hope for life to return to normal and the statistical tendency for things to *regress to the mean*. However, there is never a true, consistent state of normal, and at most, we might return to routines that are similar to, but not the same as, the time before the long-term chaos event. What people long for is not actually "normal," but rather is driven by nostalgia and traditions.

Several months into a chaos event, human elasticity diminishes—there is no "snap back" to the pre-chaos "normal." In fact, returning to normal might be undesirable, considering the expedited technological leaps that the event forced. Examples of positive changes during the most recent chaos event include things such as telemedicine, remote work, and distance learning.

Would you want to visit your doctor's office for a routine check-up that could be facilitated through the use of a tablet or app-based monitors? How about that rush hour commute? The curbside trend should never go away.

Making people come inside, go through metal detectors, check in with a receptionist. . . . Why? What emerging trends call for attention because of their disruptive potential?

The from-real-lives parables in this book tell the beyond numbers phenomena of human interaction with chaos events. Learning and using the skills discussed in this book will help readers understand human behavior during these events. More critically, it will help readers survive and even thrive during both chaos events and everyday stressors.

NOTES

1. Agel, Jerome. *The Medium is the Massage—An Inventory of Effects* (Canada: Penguin Books, 2003), 16.

2. Locke, John. *An Essay Concerning Human Understanding*, 1689, 2.9.1. https://www.gutenberg.org/files/10615/10615-h/10615-h.htm.

3. Locke, *Concerning Human Understanding*, 2.9.1.

4. Perrodin, David, P. *School of Errors: Rethinking School Safety in America* (Lanham, MD: Rowman & Littlefield, 2019), 15.

Chapter 1

Temporal Perception

THE TORUS

Adhering to a routine or a detailed schedule is one of the ways people can feel like they have some control over the world. Routines help us cope with the continual flow of decisions that face us in everyday life. They are energy-saving mechanisms that help us couple behaviors to repetitive patterns and activities, such as getting dressed in the morning. We have free will over picking out our outfits, but the left sock always goes on first, right?

Turn off the alarm clock, wiggle your feet into fuzzy slippers, poke through the closet, lay out toiletries on the vanity top, brew a cup of coffee, and swipe through the headlines.

Thirty minutes later you are off to work—which, until 2020, was a longer commute than strolling to your laptop in the living room.

Torus theory is the ingrained human behavior of feverishly pursuing a similar condition of being. We want today to be like yesterday and tomorrow to be like today.

People vehemently resist the formless disorder that is chaos. In fact, chaos is natural and liberates us so that we can consider nonlinear options, opening a window to a different way of doing things.

But humans refuse to embrace chaos, whether it manifests as a fire devouring a medieval cathedral or a shooter rampaging through the hallways of a school. We fight it. We seek to reboot to a state of pre-chaos. This seems right; it feels necessary. It's badged as healing or as preservation by our reptilian brain. But that can be a myopic and incomplete way of doing things.[1]

Thus, there is a dark side to routine. Too much could lock us into seeing ourselves on our inner tube as our only place of safety, which is the last place you want to be when riptides of chaos tear at the human condition. Two things contribute to locking us within our torus of comfort: anchoring heuristics and normalcy bias.

Macron's Pledge—The Anchoring Heuristic

An anchoring heuristic is the human tendency to accept and rely on the first piece of information received before making a decision. That first piece of information is the anchor and sets the tone.

On April 15, 2019, against an ember-glowing backdrop, France's President Emmanuel Macron vowed to the world that France would rebuild the smoldering Notre Dame cathedral.

> Yet, at that stage, he had not been informed of the scope of the damage, the potential for the building to collapse, or importantly, the root cause of the blaze. Did anyone question at that stage whether it even made sense to rebuild the cathedral? Macron delivered what people wanted to hear but not what they needed to hear, i.e., the message was that "everything will return to normal."[2]

In other words, he recognized that people were terrified to consider an altered torus and anchored them to believe that the cathedral would be rebuilt.

Normalcy Bias—Just-in-Time Competency

Normalcy bias refers to an attitude that is entered when facing a disaster. People with a normalcy bias have difficulties reacting to something they have not experienced before. They also tend to interpret warnings in the most optimistic way possible, seizing on any ambiguities to infer a less serious situation.

According to *New York Times* bestselling author and disaster researcher Amanda Ripley, "Whether they're in shipwrecks, hurricanes, plane crashes or burning buildings, people in peril experience remarkably similar stages. And the first one—even in the face of clear and urgent danger—is almost always a period of intense disbelief."[3]

Normalcy-biased people are resolute in their belief of the elasticity of the torus, when they should believe in their own judgment and discretion to assess situations and act in their best interest. (Note: You will learn more about the stay-put power of normalcy bias when we dissect the Gatlinburg wildfires later on in this chapter.)

THE ETERNAL PRESENT

Packing for a long weekend at a mountain cabin likely includes a few Band-Aids in a suitcase, and maybe some bug spray or sunblock. After a long drive far from home and up into the mountains, most people are worried about little more than if the cabin's Wi-Fi signal is strong. Entering the cabin, they scan the bulletin board by the door for the Wi-Fi password and are struck, for the first time, by the numerous snapshots of bears pinned to the cork.

In each shot, anywhere from one to four bears are seen roaming about the grounds near the cabin. There is one by the trash cans. Two sniffing the grill. Four near the picnic tables and even one climbing the tree near the deck with the hot tub. Sure, the website advised there were bears in the area, but who was expecting this?

The kids run back out to the car to continue unloading luggage and groceries, but now mom tells them to wait for dad. She asks her husband what kind of bears those are and what they should do if they see one? Dad shrugs and hurries out to supervise the car's unpacking since it is getting late and the sun is setting. Mom watches from a window and googles "bear attacks" on her phone without bothering to log in to the cabin Wi-Fi.

For most of us, our normalcy bias is calibrated to a level of comfort and convenience that is itself a luxury that would have been unfathomable for most of human history. It has become the water most of us swim in by default, and we expect those standards wherever we go.

It is as if, conceptually, we float on our inner tube in the center of a rotating diorama of locations and entertainments that may change our scenery or options, but never our safety or security. A serious consideration of risk is necessary for others, such as bush pilots in the Arctic or adventurers in the Amazon, but not for a parent who works in an office or a family on vacation in the mountains.

Or is it?

No matter how fast we receive information, sometimes it is not fast enough. This assertion holds true downtown as well as out in the suburbs, and even more so in places like remote, sparsely populated mountain resorts.

In town, a flat tire or dead battery is more of an inconvenience than a crisis, and even if you have never changed a tire or used jumper cables, you can look it up on your smartphone or employ the same phone to call a tow truck.

Low urgency situations can be easily sorted out with some thumb-typing or a quick call. The same does not apply to situations involving a higher level of urgency. Imagine searching the Internet for "what to do when a bear charges" when you first notice the bear on the trail up ahead. Or looking up "treat water moccasin bite" while you are kneeling beside your spouse in a shallow stream beside the snake you just stomped to death but not before it bit them just above the ankle.

What is the fastest way down the mountain? Where is the nearest hospital or clinic? Should I dial 911? And how is the cell service on the side of that mountain, pardner?

At times like these, the speed at which we receive information relevant to the situation will never be fast enough. Yet, we assume that our mobile devices and fast download speeds will make up for our lack of foresight, training, and experience. Yes, we are familiar with flashlights, but very few of us have marked a hiking trail, applied a tourniquet, or unfolded a single asset of a multi-tool pocketknife.

The tendency now is to prepare for everything to go just as we expect it to. We thereby magnify the risks we sidestep considering as though acknowledging the risks will somehow make them come to pass. We lapse into superstitious avoidance and roll the dice.

A little light self-sufficiency goes a long way and does not make you a doomsday prepper hunkering down in the abandoned missile silo you bought to ride out the apocalypse. Some extra food and medicine on-hand during times when so many people urge limited contact with others means fewer trips to the store and, therefore, less exposure to the threat of a contagion. Is that a bad thing?

Likewise, is learning about risks and how to mitigate or manage them before a vacation to a remote, rural wilderness area a good idea, even though it might be something of a buzzkill? Or more pointedly: will relying on "just-in-time competency" help or hurt during an immediate crisis in which time slows down, stands still, and runs out when we need to act quickly but do not know what to do or how to do it?

At that point, your smartphone's ultimate utility may be for locating your lifeless body via GPS or capturing a blurry shot of a charging bear as time stands still for you, for good.

Stopping a bear attack? There is no app for that.

GOOD MORNING, YOU'VE BEEN SORTED: ESSENTIAL OR NONESSENTIAL

Is your work essential? Everyone's work is essential to their own life. Work gives people the money that puts food on the dinner table. Work pays for everything from braces to vacations to college education. Work fills days and can even offer purpose.

But in March 2020, when a novel coronavirus disease reached America, essential was no longer up for self-designation. In most states, "essential" was a status assigned by state governors. Whether you held "essential" status decided whether or not your workplace was open. If not, your livelihood was on hold.

There were no checks and balances. This situation was an emergency. This situation was a global pandemic. If the governor of your state said you were nonessential and the media agreed, who were you, as an individual business owner or employee with bills coming in, to say any differently?

What Becomes of the Nonessential?

If some workplaces were essential, others had to be nonessential. Overnight, the default settings switched. Until that moment, you took your ability to work for granted. You decided where to go and when. Then, one day, you turned on the TV, and it was the *New Normal*.

If your work was not "essential," and therefore not allowed during the early pandemic, you were instructed to "stay home and stay safe," and collect unemployment until further notice. Watch for the next push alert at the next press conference. Watch the next press conference to hear about your livelihood.

To stay home was to stay safe, and in order to leave home, you needed either a specific reason or a permission slip, marking your work as "essential." News of the *New Normal* came in fast. Those press conferences were not of theoretical interest, as a good citizen. They were talking about your future.

Will work be open on Friday? Church on Sunday? Will your children be in school? Will the unemployment office answer when you call? Your life was now governed by a different set of questions than it had been just a month before the pandemic. You had no say-so in the answers. No amount of data or safety protocols offered in your defense mattered, and besides, to whom would you appeal? This situation was an emergency. This situation was a global pandemic.

The lists themselves seemed to make little sense. "Essential" was stocking shelves at a liquor store or answering phones at a marijuana dispensary.[4] "Nonessential" was a medical office that did breast cancer screenings. Liquor stores and dispensaries remained open, while churches and schools shut their doors.

Suddenly, opening the doors of a restaurant or a gym or a barbershop was a radical, illegal act, liable to bring the scorn of one's neighbors. Neighborly scorn was the best-case scenario. Worst-case scenario was when those who bucked restrictions were crushed by the full weight of the state, which manifested in tickets, padlocks, court orders, and even jail time.

In the eyes of the state, and the press, a nonessential business opening its doors was irresponsible. It was something only selfish scofflaws would do. Among the earliest targets of the closures, and the last to be welcomed back into the community of businesses, were gyms, hair stylists, and restaurants (figure 1.1).

One of the "non-essentials" who pushed back was Karl Manke, an Owosso, Michigan barber, then seventy-seven. When the State of Michigan declared his work nonessential and his still-open workplace illegal, Manke kept showing up, kept opening his doors, and kept cutting hair.

In May 2020, the Karl Manke Barber Shop in Owosso came to the state's attention. The state's disproportionate response brought Manke to the nation's attention and appearances on Fox News and the Glenn Beck radio show soon followed. Off-camera, Michigan State Police served papers demanding the barbershop close, and the state health director declared it an "imminent danger."

The state was using its full weight to declare a specific business unsafe.[5] Manke had announced the reopening publicly, rather than opening his doors quietly. In a blog post, Manke wrote: "There comes a time when all of us must take responsibility for our own actions. I believe my time has arrived."[6]

Manke hid in plain sight, welcoming in reporters for interviews and continuing to cut hair in open defiance of the state. The state came down hard,

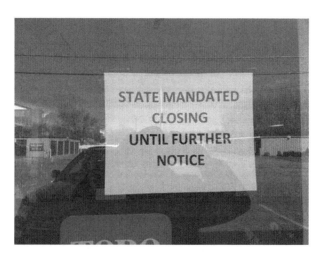

Figure 1.1 Sign on Door at Small Engines Business in Wisconsin. *Credit David P. Perrodin.*

trying to shutter the business with court orders and even going after Manke's barber license.

In June, barbershops were allowed to reopen, but Manke was still under official orders to remain closed. It took the Michigan Supreme Court to vacate that order allowing Manke to operate legally, like every other barbershop.[7]

In October, with the case over, Manke's pandemic violations were dropped altogether, as the law Governor Gretchen Whitmer cited in the emergency order was ruled unconstitutional by the Michigan Supreme Court. But Manke's legal troubles were not over just yet. The state is a powerful adversary. And it was still going after his barber's license.[8]

In March 2021, more than a year after the pandemic started, and ten months after Karl the Barber made national news headlines, the Michigan Board of Barber Examiners fined Manke $9,000 for various violations.

Among those violations, according to *The Detroit News*: "Carrying a comb in his pocket, accumulating hair and neck guards on the floor at the barber shop, and participating in a May 20 haircut protest on the Michigan Capitol steps in May."[9]

Manke's attorney, David Kallman, said his client would appear, and alleged that the state's actions were retaliatory. "This just demonstrates the pettiness and vindictiveness of the state in all of their actions against Karl over the last year," Kallman said.[10]

The lesson of Karl the Barber is that fights for one's livelihood can be won, but not without cost. Hiding in plain sight and taking an avalanche of consequence made the public more sympathetic. If an elderly man trying to make the mortgage payment is an imminent danger, then what are the rest of us?

"Essentially" at Risk

Businesses denied "essential" status fought hard for it in court, or found other ways to make themselves useful. In chapter 4 of this book, you will meet Aaron Sawyer, owner of Redline VR, a virtual reality club in Chicago.

With his business far down on the government's list, and bills coming in, Sawyer pivoted, opening Redline VR as an office space to those looking for a change from the endless busyness of working from home. The *New Normal* blurred those lines, and leaving home for an office environment helped some Chicagoans redraw the boundaries between home and work.

But for some workers, "essential" status was not an honor. What "essential" really meant was, they were the people onto whom society offloaded its risk. While the nonessential were allowed to "stay home and stay safe," Zooming online to their jobs in pajama bottoms or collecting unemployment that paid as well as a middle-class job, the essential workers were made to soldier through it. The essential workers were put face-to-face daily with a public that, in March 2020, was told that wearing masks does not help.[11]

While some were fighting to work, others were fighting for the right to be deemed nonessential, and to stay home. In suburban Detroit, a handful of workers at an Amazon fulfillment center walked out and staged a protest.[12] Meanwhile, the Michigan Infrastructure and Transportation Association, the trade association for construction workers, asked that Governor Gretchen Whitmer deem construction projects "nonessential."[13]

Employees at several businesses, including the grocery delivery firm Instacart, staged one-day walkouts.[14] Many received hazard pay, belatedly, covering a portion of their work during the pandemic. And many have argued publicly that the money did not match the risk.

One essential group hit especially hard by COVID-19 was law enforcement. Police who patrol streets, safeguard courtrooms, and secure jails cannot work from home. Indeed, when people broke government-ordered COVID-19 restrictions, it was often the police who responded.

The Detroit Police Department saw massive quarantines during the pandemic. At one point, 500 sworn officers were forced onto the sidelines, either sick themselves or in close, recent contact with someone who was. Even Police Chief James Craig fell ill briefly.[15]

During the pandemic, Detroit police wrote 1,732 tickets for violating COVID-19 restrictions, only to have 1,600-plus tossed, because the police (through Governor Whitmer's orders) had no legal authority to issue them. How many officers got sick writing tickets that were eventually thrown out? Just how "essential" was that work?

Early on in the pandemic, Charlie LeDuff, a Pulitzer Prize–winning reporter, found an odd juxtaposition between the "essential" jobs and those that carry prestige and high pay. "There goes the garbage man," LeDuff wrote. "He is essential. Without him, trash piles up, vermin come, disease grows."[16] As dirty as that work is, LeDuff wrote, it compared favorably to that of "the swells, the stockbrokers, the bankers, the lobbyists, the lawyers." By contrast, those formerly elite, "[t]oday," LeDuff wrote, "they seem, essentially, the problem."[17]

Just as the definition of "essential" and "nonessential" workers shifted under the weight of a pandemic, so too, has our perception of information relative to the passage of time.

PHYSICS OF TIME

Imagine being a subsistence farmer in the late 1700s. You need some help building a fence, so after church one Sunday, you make arrangements with a neighbor to meet you next Tuesday on the property line you share. You both agree to meet at noon, and since neither of you owns a watch, "noon" is determined by the position of the sun in the sky.

You arrive at "noon" to find your neighbor napping in the shade of a large tree. You call to him as you approach and once he gets up, you find out he had been there for some time. Thirty minutes, perhaps. Maybe forty-five. Either way, it is a nonissue as neither of you owns a watch nor has any expectation that your home clocks are synchronized. So your mutual expectation is that one of you will arrive in advance of the other and will wait since observing the noon sun from different locations lacks precision.

This patience and resignation are effects of dealing with time and travel as a physical constraint. Smoke signals and semaphore aside, communications between two distant points can only be accomplished by messenger through travel. This restriction strongly affects thinking and expectations.

Benefiting from twenty-first-century smartphones and map apps, most of us would regard waiting forty-five minutes for someone to arrive at a meeting to imply some kind of accident or an act of rudeness. This attitude is because technology provides communication at great precision and speed. We are not nearly as limited as our cohorts in the 1700s; therefore, our expectations are much different.

> The pace of information processing has undoubtedly increased, but the perception of that speed is not new. Late 19th century Europeans had a similar sense of rapidly changing forms of communication, commerce, and development as a result. So while the size, speed, and type of increase in technology precipitates change, the perceptions of those changes matter as well.[18]

In the eighteenth century, you did not expect to have advance notice or the ability to visit your family or friends in another state when they got sick; you expected to hear that they had been ill for some time, and then died. By contrast, most of us expect to hear of illnesses or accidents within minutes of the event or diagnosis regardless of where in the world our friend or loved one lives.

The velocity (speed of information in a direction) has changed. Information directed specifically to each of us is arriving faster, and with greater accuracy, than any time in human history.

Thus, we walk around with the expectation of speed and precision of information. We rely on it. It is our default mindset, so when we experience a disruption of this conditioned expectation of immediate information, many of us equate this with significant system failure or breakdown, whether such is actually the case or not. It feels like the case because we regard it as a significant departure from the norm. And indeed, in some ways, it is.

Smoky Mountains—The Collapse of Physical Time

Consider the wildfires that killed 14 people and destroyed nearly 20,000 acres in the Pigeon Forge and Gatlinburg areas of the Great Smoky Mountains of Eastern Tennessee in November and December 2016.[19] More specifically, imagine being among the residents and vacationers in the Gatlinburg, Tennessee area attempting to flee down the mountainside at night, in the dark, in some cases encountering downed trees and abandoned automobiles blocking roadways, while walls of flame consuming trees and underbrush rapidly approach the road from both sides.

"At 8:30 p.m. on November 28, 2016, high winds and roaring flames disabled cell towers, melted fiber-optic cables, disrupted digital radio signals and shut down phone lines. Backup systems and protocols failed."[20] Everything cut out in an instant.

Such is a perfect storm of problems, and one of these is a communications problem. The deeper and higher one gets into the mountains, the more complicated navigation becomes. Even roads in many resort areas can be narrow, winding, poorly lit at night, and challenging to navigate under normal conditions.

Road signs are sometimes missing or damaged due to storms or driver error. During storms and natural disasters, power poles may fall across roads, hindering passage and exposing travelers to dangerous live wires. Cellular service can be spotty, and GPS coordinates less precise or poorly synced to twisting networks of roads, some of which turn out to be dead-ends or service roads that lead one deeper into the mountains instead of down to the communities below.

Smartphone map applications in these areas often prove unreliable under normal circumstances when the most pressing problem is getting down the mountain and into town before the pizza place closes.

This same unreliability during a raging wildfire can introduce the gravest of situations to residents and visitors alike in more remote areas where our elaborate communication systems and technology cannot overcome the challenges posed by the physical realities of geography, darkness, and the very real possibility of death by smoke inhalation and fire.

Two men living in the area experienced this reality when a single burning ember fell into their yard and made them realize they had perhaps misjudged the fire's proximity and degree of threat. Perhaps they expected more in the way of official communications and warning, or someone to take charge and make a decision, but none preceded the smoke, the orange glow in the sky, or, ultimately, that ember in the brothers' yard.[21]

The National Institute of Standards and Technology (NIST) found that "less than a quarter of surveyed residents received any type of warning or had prepared an evacuation plan for their household."[22]

Emily Walpole, a NIST scientist who studied the incident, uncovered a perplexing finding in her analysis of the multiday fire. "It's possible that you get used to smelling smoke and it basically lulls you into a false sense of security . . . the fire could be miles away and be producing smoke."[23]

Likewise, some resorts and vacationers in the area ignored the nearby threat until it was almost too late. "It seemed that people expected that if a large wildfire requiring evacuation was going to happen, they would be told. Instead, many had to find out on their own."[24]

Resorts closed, issuing eleventh-hour evacuation orders as their hope that the fires would spare their area was extinguished, while the fire was not. One such couple relates how it was not until they texted a picture of encroaching fire to their firefighter son—who replied for them to get out of the area immediately—that their own perception of their immediate situation changed.[25]

In the case of the brothers spurred to action by the appearance of the ember in their yard—a sort of "shot across the bow" from the fire itself—they quickly packed some items into a pickup truck and fled down the mountainside, only to be stopped by a downed telephone pole across the road.

The obstruction forced them to improvise and find another route down while propane tanks exploded nearby. So close, in fact, that they could feel the heat pulse in the truck as they breathed the smoke wafting in through the vents.

During descent, they encountered a car stopped in the middle of the road blocking it. The driver, an elderly gentleman who could not see because of the darkness and thick smoke, followed the brothers' taillights down the mountain. It seemed to be his last option.[26]

Out of time, lost, confused, sensory-deprived, and not only cut off from any help but also from the ability to communicate due to nearby cell towers being destroyed or overwhelmed, the elderly man was fortunate that the brothers had been forced in his direction. Others were not so fortunate, and never made it down.[27]

Many of us rely so heavily on "smart" devices on a daily basis when hell is not breaking loose. We have trained ourselves to assume that the technology that allows us to receive the information we need to navigate our home turf on a typically uneventful day will always work because it always has worked. This assumption is our torus, our normalcy bias.

Our baseline, daily offloading to our technology has allowed us to adopt a less-than-critical mindset toward technology. It simply never occurs to us that our devices and systems could fail to give us "just-in-time" control on a dark, smoke-filled night navigating maze-like roadways in life-threatening conditions on a burning mountainside.

The eighteenth-century neighbors who just needed to get "close enough" have evolved into contemporary adventurers who throw caution to the wind by outsourcing competency and offloading knowledge to satellites and cloud networks because "close enough" is no longer good enough. After all, we live in an age when physical challenges are just a matter of solving technical problems using our portable, powerful communications and computing devices that provide us the precision we demand, the precision we may even need to save our life one day.

Driving in circles in a maze of narrow roads on a burning mountainside at night without directions? There is usually an app for that.

PSYCHOLOGICAL TIME

In addition to physical effects, our perception of time also has the ability to effectuate psychological consequences. Locke identified chaos' ability to separate us from time—as we fill our minutes by actions we believe will ease our pain and not necessarily solve our problems. Time also seems to change speed depending upon our age.

As we get older, we have fewer new experiences and the world around us becomes more and more familiar. Our inner tube still floats, but closer to the shore. We only float in waters we know well, and that is acceptable to us. That amicable, familiar relationship can make us appear reclusive or even in the early stages of mental decline.

This phenomenon is depicted in the following account provided to the author of this book by a prominent mental health expert.

Your Dad's Losing It

This recollection is based on a transcribed conversation in 2021 between the author and "Olivia," a mental health expert who prefers to remain anonymous.[28]

"Your Dad's losing it," she said, when I picked up the phone that otherwise unexceptional day nine months into the COVID-19 lockdown.

You would think Mom—a geriatric nurse for sixty years—would have a gentler way of discussing dementia with her children. The previous day, my father had her feverishly searching every channel for his favorite team's NCAA basketball game, without success, and much to both of their frustration.

"Punch it up again!" he shouted—his way of asking both his wife and four adult children to "google" something on their smartphones. He knew the team played at 1:00; he knew what channel they were on; he knew their opponent, their record, the stats of the key players, the rank of both teams, even the hometowns and high schools of the majority of the team.

As a lifelong newsman and sportscaster, he spent his career researching and gathering this minutia so that he could provide the most color while calling various sports over the rural area's oldest radio station waves. Whether pounding away on his oldfangled Smith-Corona, in the airtight radio booth where he spent his forty-two-year career, or in the chair in front of the TV where he spent all his days now, his memory was a gift that kept giving well into his eighties.

At eighty-five, and nearly deaf, he had lost a bit of recall, but none of the fervor with which he called the games—much to his children's and grandchildren's delight.

I had been regularly visiting my parents on Tuesdays for over a year when this happened. My brother went on Sundays, and my eldest sister on some Fridays and Saturdays.

After hearing my mom's concerns, I dutifully sent a sibling group text stating, "Dad is losing time and day orientation. We may need to put some accommodations in place over the holidays." I then "punched up" Hammacher Schlemmer and added the "Easy Read Full Disclosure Clock" to my cart. The clock gave the time and additional orientation information (i.e., December 15, 2:00 Tuesday, *afternoon*). Problem solved. I would give it to him at Christmas and tell him we just needed a better clock in the living room. No reason to mention the loss of anything.

Routine. Orientation. Accommodations. These are things people, young and old, depend on every day. But what if routines are upset by a mass chaos event? What if orientation never matters, because you do not leave your home for months at a time? Maybe due to an event, perhaps due to being a lifelong hermit now freed of the few social responsibilities you once had (in this case, church on Sundays, weekly Friday night shrimp dinner at Culvers, a monthly haircut, and a quarterly trip to Fleet Farm).

If no day requires appointments or necessary social interactions, as is the case of many elderly retirees, how will you (and why do you need to) know what day of the month or even day of the week it is?

In this case, my father explained, it was not his "losing it" that was to blame, but rather his wife's "new crazy schedule," or actually, the lack thereof. Without her getting up at certain times, dressing certain ways, and coming and going on a strict schedule, combined with his complete release from social expectations due to months of lockdown, he had lost orientation to the day and even month. It was no longer important. And it was not due to dementia, concluded Olivia.[29]

Young and old alike have experienced some version of psychological time dilation, defined by *Merriam-Webster* dictionary as "a slowing of time in accordance with the theory of relativity that occurs in a system in motion relative to an outside observer."[30]

If you had a teenager or were a teenager during the initial weeks after the chaos of the COVID-19 lockdown, the first three weeks may have felt more like three years. The inability of teens and even younger tweens to define who they were and how time was passing through acts of socialization left many anxious, unmoored, and drifting.

TIME DILATION

To understand time dilation in children, become familiar with the simple figure of a train, a child, and an adult. The train is collectively representative of the COVID-19 pandemic. Unseen are the coupled cars of civil unrest, economic strife, and shattered relationships rattling beyond its tender. The adult is equidistant from the train and from the child. The child is standing on the tracks facing the nose of the locomotive (figure 1.2).

The locomotive is traveling at a constant speed. Its velocity is determined by the tracks.

From the perspective of the child, the locomotive seems to accelerate as it closes distance to him. This situation is new and happening quickly. His mind frantically attempts to pattern stimuli overpowering his senses. The engine engulfs his field of vision. Wooden ties under his feet rumble and then pulse as they take on the tonnage of the iron horse.

Moments later, the boy's hair ripples back and his shirt sleeves flap as the locomotive displaces more air. Turbulence. A torrent of clangs, hisses, and booms swallow the boy. The locomotive blasts its horn—again and again . . . Deafening. Overwhelming!

From the perspective of the man, the train is steady and not accelerating. He will endure glancing consequences of its approach and passing, a blast of silted, exhaust-thick wind, a startle as the horn lights up his amygdala, an area of the brain that contributes to emotional processing, sending a distress signal to the hypothalamus which immediately signals the adrenal glands to pump adrenaline into the bloodstream.

Heart rate and blood pressure spike. Hairs stand up on his neck. He is stressed, yet he does not misdoubt the train's velocity and that, barring an unforeseen event, he stands upon safe ground.

The child's brain may be sending the same "fight, flight, or freeze" readiness signals, but the child is unlikely to be able to put the sensory inputs aside and make a rational decision about how easily he could move out of the way. Time, in his frame of reference, is moving too fast.

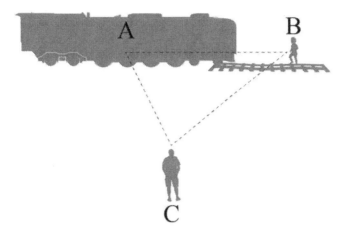

Figure 1.2 Time Dilation for Children. *Credit David P. Perrodin and Aimee K. DiStefano;* OpenClipart-Vectors, train-locomotive #157837, n.d., Pixabay. Free for commercial use, no attribution required. https://pixabay.com/vectors/train-locomotive-railway-157837/; OpenClipart-Vectors, rails-railway #155636, n.d., Pixabay. Free for commercial use, no attribution required. https://pixabay.com/vectors/rails-railway-tracks-trackage-mine -155636/; Gordon Johnson, child-baby #1769717, n.d., Pixabay. Free for commercial use, no attribution required. https://pixabay.com/vectors/child-baby-toddler-infant-kid -1769717/; Lulian Mindrila, silhouettes-men #1283534, n.d., Pixabay. Free for commer-cial use, no attribution required. https://pixabay.com/vectors/silhouettes-men-man-man -silhouette-1283534/.

They're Digging Out the Playground   *← rumor mill*

"They're digging out the playground," announced a defeated nine-year-old girl. The breaking news arrived by email from a classmate, via a friend, who believed that they saw city workers dismantling the playground either yester-day or sometime this morning.

Exasperated, she looked away and frowned. First, school was closed and then she was not allowed to visit her friends. Neighborhood bike rides were truncated to loops on the driveway, and now the playground was added to the growing list of banished things.

Her father assured her that the playgrounds were still there, at the schools, across the city, and aside from being snarled in yellow police tape, nothing had changed. Nothing, except official-looking signs citing number-jumble statutes justifying why the playgrounds looked like scary crime scenes.

Still, the daughter could not think beyond the dystopian illustrations convincingly shared by her network of keyed up friends. Her father knew he could talk until the cows came home and it would not make a lick of difference.

"Put on your coat and bring your mask," he said as he tucked the camera tripod under his arm. "We're going to check out what's happening in town," declared the father with a hint of adventure in his voice and a tinge of safer-at-home defiance hubris in this nonessential outing.

The father understood that if you are going through something that is bad, it is best to try to find a purpose in it. Even if this is a bit of mental trickery, it will help you to see you through. And in that moment, the father and daughter set out on what would be the first of thirteen short videos recorded in the next four months to capture "what was happening in town."

The videos would serve as an archive, explained the father. "Years from now, you'll be able to show your family what it was like to be a kid during the pandemic." In choosing his words, he framed the situation as transitory—this was somewhat like the pass by of a comet.

They set out to observe the surroundings and were all at once less focused on the yellow police tape whipping in the cold March winds and the sad, dark imagery of a closed playground (figure 1.3).

Instead, their attention centered on positioning the camera to capture video and rehearsing impromptu news reporter-ish narratives that identified locations, dates, what was present, and how it had changed from what was there before. It would not be perfect, as the times were not perfect, and they would fix things in postproduction.

This ongoing documentation activity helped reduce the dilation of time for the girl and contributed to mitigating the sense of chaos she experienced from all of the changes to her routine.

Young People and Chaos

When assessing the velocity of information, young people will perceive it differently than older people. They judge that events happen slower and last longer relative to their adult counterparts.

This difference in perception is due to the time dilation effect that occurs when events involving an object coming toward you last longer in psychological time than an event with the same object being stationary. Some of this is simply attempting to process fast-moving, unfamiliar information and match it to something we have been through before.

An adult's thinking is faster and is able to process more, find more patterns, and grapple with abstract concepts—such as the rationing of care, the logistics of testing millions of people, or ethics of classifying someone as essential. Some of this is due to brain development, as well as just simply more experience with making it through chaotic times.

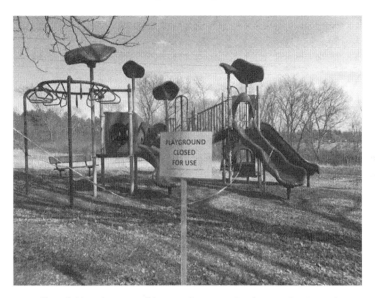

Figure 1.3   Closed City Playground in March 2020. *Credit David P. Perrodin.*

Whereas kids can get overwhelmed by the deluge of information and the subsequent waves that knock them off their torus and prevent them from escaping the chaos event. They are told what to do—already the state of being a kid—and now the messaging seeps through starchy face masks.

Time seems to slow down when we are exposed to new environments and experiences. Children have more "new" experiences than adults and will spend more time processing information versus patterning it. The moment can have a whirlpool effect on kids, swirling them deeper instead of unobtrusively twirling them downstream to their next adventure.

Another way to think about this is by putting yourself in the mindset of a forty-year-old person experiencing a hurricane for the first time. You would likely feel anxious and unprepared versus a counterpart who has lived their entire life in Cape Hatteras, North Carolina—a city affected by 110 hurricanes since 1871.[31]

There is also a proportional aspect to time. As we get older, each period of time constitutes a smaller proportion of our life as a whole. A nine-year-old in 2020 lived 10 percent of his life during the epoch of COVID-19/Civil Unrest. His fifty-year-old grandparent, in comparison, experienced only 2 percent of his life during the same period of time.

Thus, the proportionality of time and time dilation can have a significant impact on young people and children. One way to counter the effects of time dilation is to become more situationally aware.

SITUATIONAL AWARENESS: GATHERING
INDICATORS WITH JOE DOLIO

For general public safety after 9/11, Americans were encouraged to be more aware of their environment. According to the U.S. Department of Homeland Security, situational awareness is knowing and understanding what is happening around you.[32]

For instance, we use situational awareness daily when we see an unattended suitcase at an airport or when walking to our car at night while being alert to dangers. Situational awareness involves using input from all of our senses to comprehend the current situation and to anticipate risks.

An indicator is a piece of information that tends to point toward a particular conclusion. You use indicators every day, yet just do not call them that. Imagine you are walking down a hallway, and you see Bob walking toward you. Bob's shoulders are slumped, and he has a frown on his face. Your first thoughts are that Bob is not in a good mood. You arrived at this conclusion by using the indicators that Bob displayed.

Another example that we all use without knowing is when we have been indoors, in the office all day, and then someone walks in, dripping wet. Invariably, our first question aloud to that person is, "Oh, is it raining outside?" The person's wet clothing is an indicator.

When addressing the velocity of information and talking about crisis response, indicators are an important weather gauge and a method either to prove or disprove a general trend or conclusion. When you are trying to determine if it is raining outside, you look out the window. You are looking for wet ground, rain on the window, and water dripping from things outside. These are all indicators.

Gathering indicators is nothing more than observing what is going on around you and taking a very short pause to make an educated guess about what is most likely happening now, and what is likely to happen in the next few minutes. Antecedent indicators prime your calculations of response options. Paying attention to those indicators will help safely navigate any situation.

Joe Dolio is a U.S. Marine Corps Veteran with over twenty years in corporate security investigations as a Certified Fraud Examiner and Certified Forensic Interviewer.[33] He is a KyoSaNim (Instructor) and Second-Degree Black Belt in Tang Soo Do. Dolio's training and experience give him a unique perspective on identifying indicators during times of chaos or crisis.

In the late fall of 2020, Dolio saw signs appear at the local grocery store limiting quantities of fresh chicken purchases. Knowing that this could indicate a potential shortage, he made an unplanned purchase of the maximum amount, in response to the indicator.

After making that purchase, Dolio conducted an analysis to look for additional indicators to support or refute the position that a potential shortage was looming. He decided to look for: (1) similar or the same signs at additional stores; (2) indicators from member checks; and (3) media stories about chicken processing/farming issues.

After deciding on these, Dolio went to work to examine them. A quick trip to other stores confirmed that purchase-limit signs were up throughout the area. However, a member check call (calling someone else in a different area of Michigan) revealed that there were no signs elsewhere, just in the local area. A review of media showed that there was a COVID-19 outbreak at a local cold-storage facility that provided fresh chicken products throughout the area.

By verifying these indicators and through member checks, Dolio learned that the problem was localized and, therefore, most likely very temporary, as major grocers would quickly line up alternate supply lines.

The process is simple: in your daily life, be on the alert for indicators of potential trouble. When you see one indicator, develop a list of what other indicators would confirm the issue, and what ones would refute it, then set out to check those indicators.

The U.S. military calls this the "Priority Information Requirements Process," or "PIR Process." The premise is that when a unit is faced with particular circumstances, courses of action are developed to respond, along with a list of PIRs that would confirm which course of action is best according to priority indicators.

You already do this in daily life, likely without realizing it. What do you do when you are driving down the freeway and look ahead, seeing long lines of stopped traffic, and there is an exit immediately to your right?

You observe the indicator of stopped traffic for miles pointing toward the course of action of you exiting the freeway to drive around the obstruction. Once off the stopped freeway, you query your GPS device for more information (indicators) to help you find a route around the blockage.

When we are consumed and distracted with the endless attention-getters in life, we fail to recognize or actively scan for indicators. Bombarded with information from electronic stimuli, and additionally confounded by normalcy bias, we reduce our ability to discern the truth.

One example of this came in early 2020, as the COVID-19 pandemic began. There were nonstop news stories about the people rushing out to buy toilet paper. There were other people who laughed them off and said, "Look at these silly people rushing out to buy toilet paper!" Within days, some of those same people who mocked the others were online begging for a source for toilet paper.

It is a phenomenon that can be explained and avoided. It began with a few people panic-buying. Then others saw this and said, "Well, that seems crazy, but I had better get some before the lunatics buy it all," which then snowballed until the supply was gone, and a true shortage was created.

It is very easy to laugh at or discount indicators, but this simple, low-risk example points to how easily bad things can happen when you do not analyze the second- and third-order effects of human thinking and behavior. Dolio teaches this in his security awareness classes.

Most people look at indicators and see the "first-order" effect of "crazed people hoarding toilet paper." The second-order effect was other people deciding that they had better buy some, too, because the "panic-stricken" were going to buy it all if they did not. The third-order effect was the widespread toilet paper shortage of 2020. It is interesting to note that the collective memory often only mentions the third-order effect or the indicator's eventual outcome, for example, COVID-19 caused a toilet paper shortage.

Another example was the Black Lives Matter (BLM) gatherings in the summer of 2020. When they began, the first-order effect was a show of unity across many groups against police misconduct. As other people got involved who were not committed to the originators' peaceful protest philosophy, the second-order effects became violence, property damage, and fear.

The ultimate third-order effect was an increase in distrust among many groups, which was the exact opposite of the original intent. That progression is an example of how taking action at the first observation of an indicator—in this case, removing or better controlling violent instigators—could have helped prevent the progression to negative tertiary order effects.

In Metro Detroit, the local BLM leadership observed this and took immediate action, and as a result, Detroit did not see the level of violence that other parts of the country did. In the first few days, agitators were spotted and BLM quickly pushed them out of their groups.

While other protest groups in the area asked known agitators for help organizing security, the main BLM group refused, and then removed them from their group. As a result of a quick response to the second-order effect, by observing the indicators, peaceful BLM protesters in Detroit prevented the third-order effect.

In any crisis, observing indicators and anticipating possible second- and third-order effects will help you identify the right indicators which require a reaction. But to decide objectively on which indicators to look into, you have to recognize your biases—which we will delve into in chapter 2. In the interim, we will explore what happens when you have too much information to process.

COGNITIVE OFFLOADING

Cognitive offloading refers to our reliance on the external environment in order to reduce cognitive demand. It is why we have safety protocol flip charts and Automated External Defibrillators (AEDs) that provide us with auditory and visual cues to administer a life-saving electric shock correctly to restore someone's heart to its normal rhythm. It is not necessary to practice using the AED; you only need to know the location of the AED. The charts and instructions included with the device then allow you to use the AED properly when you need it.

That is an example of cognitive offloading; we are doing it more than ever before, and it is generally a good thing.

Cognitive offloading reduces demand on memory because it does not rely on our brains to create labyrinthian neural sequences to encode information. Previous studies have shown that allowing people to offload information can significantly improve performance on short-term and prospective memory tasks.[34]

But there is a catch. You simply cannot offload cognitive abilities and proficiency with tools in the hope that you will be able to use them competently, on-demand, without practice. "Cognitive offloading is usually considered in the case of cognitive agents that *already* possess cognitive abilities, but offload information into the environment or into their relationship with the environment."[35] Technology is relevant and powerful, but we are powerless without plain technical ability.

Information is offloaded to the Internet with expectations similar to that of a complex fire engine parked in a station. We believe it will be there when we need it, accessible, unchanged, infallible, that mice have not gnawed the hoses, and that static systems will seamlessly interface with the evolved world beyond the firehouse doors.

But what if we are prohibited from accessing information stored in the cloud? "From Belarus to Myanmar, 29 countries suspended Internet services in 2020."[36] According to a 2021 report released by *Access Now* and the #KeepItOn Coalition, Internet shutdowns prevented people in dozens of countries from working, studying, communicating, and accessing life-saving news last year.[37]

The report goes on to document that Internet shutdowns occurred during protests and conflicts. In other words, people were most likely to be separated from digital information during times of crisis. This issue might not have been as significant before smartphones when knowledge and memory shared the same space.

We might think that memory is something that happens in the head, but increasingly it is becoming something that happens with the help of agents outside the head. Benjamin Storm, Sean Stone, and Aaron Benjamin conducted experiments to determine our likelihood to reach for a computer or smartphone to answer questions. Their results were jarring.

"Remarkably, 30% of participants who previously consulted the Internet failed to even attempt to answer a single simple question from memory."[38]

We can argue that the Internet is more comprehensive, dependable, and, on the whole, faster than the imperfections of human memory. In times of a stable torus, that is true. In times of chaos, it is a gamble, both for humans and their Artificial Intelligence (AI).

Sometimes it is a winning gamble: downloaded Google maps helped the colleague of an engineer find his way through shattered, unrecognizable landmarks and obscured roads in order to reunite with his family after the 2011 Fukushima earthquake in Japan.[39] The colleague accomplished this by repositioning his attention between the smart device in his hand and the rubble at his feet.

We have all driven with our phone in our hand. And not just in our hand, but actively in use. We text, we tweet, we pick our favorite song. These days, driving is more a distraction from the phone than vice-versa.

The self-driving car is not just science fantasy anymore but publicized as a problem-solver: it frees the motorist from the road, and by eliminating human error, makes the road safer. Driving is inherently dangerous. In America in 2020, 42,060 people died in car crashes.[40]

A paper by two University of Texas researchers found that if 10 percent of the vehicles on the road were self-driving cars, there would be savings of more than thirty-seven billion dollars from lives saved, fuel savings, reduced travel time, and more.[41] The estimated benefits would exceed $447 billion if 90 percent of the vehicles on the road were self-driving.[42]

Therefore, it is *assumed* that self-driving cars will be safer, but we do not really know yet, do we? Self-driving vehicles would result in even more human cognitive offloading and even greater dependence upon the machine's sensors and algorithms to complete the task—which works fine, until it does not. Stranded on a rustic road and it is getting chilly. No problem, just ask your smart device, "How do I turn on the heat in a stranded car?"

At what point have we offloaded too much?

CONTINUOUS PARTIAL ATTENTION: LINDA STONE

It is likely that no person has died from having missed a social media post. Yet it is missing the tweet we fear, and not car crashes.

In 1997, Linda Stone, a consultant and speaker on technology and human attention, named our attempts to do two activities at once that both require cognition as "continuous partial attention."[43]

According to Stone, in 1997, everyone was talking about multitasking, but they were not differentiating between simple multitasking and complex multitasking. The phrase "continuous partial attention" (CPA) made that distinction.

CPA is complex multitasking. Differentiating is important because simple multitasking is not that stressful. Complex multitasking, or CPA, is *very* stressful. And unlike cognitive offloading, our attention cannot be outsourced to the cloud.

Stone is the creator of The Attention Project: "We can enhance or augment our attention with practices like meditation, breathwork, and exercise, diffuse it with technologies like email, texting, and social media, or alter it with pharmaceuticals," her website explains.[44] "Attention," Stone writes, "is the most powerful tool of the human spirit."[45]

Velocity is speed in a direction and the surging information torrent headed our way channels us into crisis-management mode and turns up the stress. Stone notes that CPA started long before COVID-19 and was always both at work and at home, though, in our working-from-home lives, we have significantly increased the volume.

How many lit screens do we have on our kitchen table? One or two computers? A tablet? A smartphone? A smartwatch? A Fit Bit? And do our eyes monitor each screen (and a child, and the dog) while also attempting to work on one, or more, of those screens?

How many times, while working from home, did you find yourself doing multiple brain-centric activities at once: for example, writing an email while participating in a work meeting and preparing for another meeting later? If you are a parent, your child was just a few feet away doing online school. Neither one of you has worked from home before, but now both of you do.

According to Stone, "We think we can attend to more than one thing at a time, but we really use our attention rapidly and serially."[46] Attention shifts every time you monitor your child's school day. Are they paying attention? What are they being taught, and is it accurate? What will I have to re-explain later? Is there a nuance for which a group discussion does not allow?

That is a lot of questions to juggle even if you had all day. But you do not. You have a job of your own, the one that pays the mortgage and the bill for that Wi-Fi.

Never has our attention been pulled in so many directions at once. Texting while driving was always risky, but this was also an opted-in difficulty. People brought that added difficulty on themselves.

No one chose the pandemic. No one chose for school and home and work all to take place in the same space in the same hours of the day. And yet this was our life.

In March 2017, Robert Kelly, a professor, was doing a live interview about South Korean politics on BBC News when his two children found his make-shift TV studio and invited themselves inside.[47]

Kelly told *The Guardian* that he and his wife spoke in the hallway after-ward and were stunned by what had happened. "We both assumed that was the end of my career as a talking head," Kelly said. "I thought I'd blown it in front of the whole world."[48]

Instead, the video went viral and warmed hearts. Not only was the moment cute, but it also related a modern tale of the many hats people wear in life—and how little those hats mean to children who are happy to see Mom or Dad, and do not know about any talking heads. Three years later, people were not merely relating to Robert Kelly. Now it was their own children (and pets) making cameos in video meetings.

As Stone writes on her blog, CPA is not simple multitasking.[49] Consider stirring soup while talking on the phone. While stirring soup may be auto-matic, talking on the phone is not. Talking on the phone requires cognition: listening, speaking coherently. . . . Stirring soup while talking on the phone would be considered simple multitasking. When we are trying to write an email *and* talk on the phone, we are doing two things that require cognition.

Simple multitasking: one thing is automatic and one thing requires cognition.

CPA (complex multitasking): two things or more than two things require cognition.

Stone writes: "We multitask to create more opportunity for ourselves—time to do more and time to relax more."[50] But with CPA, she states, "we're motivated by a desire to not miss anything."[51]

Stone has noticed a shift in the decision-making dynamic in the COVID-19 era. Before, she said, people would ask what they have to gain from doing an activity. Now, people ask what they have to lose from not doing it.[52]

"Will I get sick from doing this? Will this exposure cause that? What will I lose if I do not do this meeting? Rather than, what will I gain?" Stone said, in a private interview. "The big questions we're dealing with have shifted."[53]

That said, having one's toddlers interrupt a work meeting is more profes-sionally acceptable than canceling the meeting. Without the office environ-ment, the collegiality, the break room, and the stop-and-chats, work product is our only way to prove value. Especially when business receipts are down.

There will be a list made, next year, or even sooner, of the people the company has to let go. No one wants to be on it. The pandemic has brought on new and existential life anxiety: Are you doing enough? After all, Bill Shakespeare wrote *King Lear* during his plague. How did you spend yours?[54]

In a work context, the person who cancels meetings today might be the one relieved of their duties when pink slip season arrives. For that and other reasons, some people are not able to let go of the workday. "They're doing Zoom calls from morning to night," Stone said.[55]

Stone feels it is important to match the technology to the activity. "As we work from home, not every conversation requires a Zoom call," she said.[56] She has advised clients to turn work meetings into a phone call, rather than a Zoom call, "unless there's a really strong reason."[57]

Stone believes that endless Zooming can be exhausting because "there's a lot of audio and visual input."[58] Phone calls can be very effective, although Zoom makes sense for some meetings. But, she advises, consider which technology best matches the activity to reduce the risk of video-meeting burnout, or becoming "Zoombified," a term coined by altRPO CEO Sean Ofeldt.[59]

Stone noted that COVID-19 restrictions add another factor. Without social options, people have more discretionary time to use or abuse. "We're limited in who we can have physical and social contact with," Stone said, adding that "[t]his gives a lot of people a lot more time for reflection, or for projects, or to be depressed, or to follow a conspiracy theory, or to develop a new hobby."[60]

Some people baked sourdough bread.[61] Some people lost weight. Some people gained it. Others used their stimulus check to trade options in the stock market and helped take down a hedge fund for billions.[62]

But the liberation of time was never realized by many; they are working, trying to help their children through the school day, juggling household issues and fickle Wi-Fi, and it takes more time and attention than they seem to have. We will discuss Parkinson's Law—the idea that work expands to fill the time available for the task—and its implications in a later chapter.

Regardless, our ability to manage this precious resource, our attention, should not be minimized without strong consideration as it is at the heart of our quality of life. As The Attention Project warns, "In the end, though, we are fully responsible for how we choose to use this extraordinary resource."[63]

What Did You Say?

There is one important caveat with respect to the concept of CPA. How do we attend to a garbled signal? COVID-19 wreaked havoc on verbal communication. Encumbered by masks and social distancing, spoken language became more difficult when masks were introduced. "Numerous studies indicate that a mask's design and material influence speech clarity of the wearer—depending on the type of mask, sound can be decreased by 3–12 decibels."[64]

Social distancing also contributed to hearing difficulties. "Distance decreases the volume picked up by the ear. The power of sound is cut in half with every three feet of added distance, so a distance of six or more feet makes it much more difficult to pick up on spoken language."[65] Consider adults in multiethnic settings where dialects and accents are involved and CPA might altogether be dropping the signal.

TECHNOLOGY ADOPTION AND
DISINTERMEDIATION

The number of connected devices is increasing, not just because of consumers' growing thirst for mobile data, but also because of concepts such as the Internet of Things (IoT). Internet users in regional areas are also turning to wireless networks as a more cost-effective way of increasing their data rates than running fiber to the home. The radio frequency band is thus getting more crowded all the time and more technological devices are vying for our attention.

According to intelligence analysts Amerson and Meridith III:

> The rate at which technology is evolving and is absorbed into use by the population is growing exponentially. Starting with the advent of electricity in 1873, nearly 46 years passed before 25% of the U.S. population utilized this new technology. This was in large part because the speed of change from the profit-seeking standpoint of utility producers ran up against the drag of government and public infrastructure slowing the diffusion.
>
> Then, with fewer and smaller-scale changes needed to implement new technology broadly, mobile phones took only 13 years to achieve the same end, and only seven years to achieve 25% absorption of the World Wide Web within the U.S. The Apple iPhone launched in 2007, selling six million units in one year in four countries, while the iPhone 3G launched in 2008, selling ten million units in five months worldwide.[66]

Because of advances in technology, people now expect to receive their news in real time. Streaming services have also emerged as an example of how consumers now expect a personalized experience when viewing content online.

At one time, journalists merely endeavored to serve a local audience, delivering news specific to the broadcast area. This focus meant putting together a few newscasts each day that were viewed by everyone who tuned in to watch. However, technology has given businesses the ability to learn about website visitors and deliver information specifically targeted to each person's interaction with a site.

This connection between a journalist and the community they covered also provided a degree of accountability often lost with digitized national news. A critical piece of effective and accurate communication is the reliability of the person providing the information.

In the past, generals and military commanders were reliant on messengers and scouts accurately conveying information about parts of the battlefield they could not see, in order to make important strategic decisions.

A reporter traditionally did not merely report on the happenings of the community; they lived there and had professional and personal relationships with the people potentially affected by what was printed. Inaccurately covering an incident or controversy could mean more than a nasty online comment.

Depending on the size of the town and newspaper, disgruntled readers could simply pay them a visit at their office. Other potential consequences were personal confrontations, advertisers pulling ads, social alienation, and a distrust among people the reporter relied on as sources as well as friends and neighbors.

This accountability was lost as more and more reporters no longer lived or even operated in that community. The loss was even greater the larger and more nationalized the news organization became, to the point where often their only restraint, if any, has been the threat of libel and defamation lawsuits. The result is widespread mistrust.

At the same time, trust in media coverage generally has dwindled, and the day may soon come when even the most basic and simplest of information reported is treated with skepticism. Ironically, that skepticism may provide new opportunities for journalists to regain public trust.

In 2017, commercial airline pilot Juan Browne received acclaim for producing more than fifty videos of the Oroville Dam failure in Northern California. He flew his private plane over the site to capture video, monitored publicly available water inflow/outflow data, made models in his den to illustrate the features of the dam and spillway, and went to the site to talk with workers with the Department of Water Resources and Kiewit Infrastructure Company.[67]

What is roller-compacted concrete and how was it placed at the upper chute of the spillway? Juan has a video on that. We will learn more about Juan and the citizen-as-journalist when we examine Face Validity in chapter 2 of this book.

NOTES

1. Perrodin, David P., "Investigating to an Absolute Conclusion." *Crisis Response Journal* 14, no. 4 (October 2019): 56.

2. Perrodin, *Absolute Conclusion*, 56.

3. Ripley, Amanda. "How to Get Out Alive." Time, April 25, 2005. http://content .time.com/time/magazine/article/0,9171,1053663,00.html.

4. Schroyer, John. "US Markets That Have Allowed Marijuana Businesses to Remain Open During Coronavirus Pandemic Stay-At-Home Orders." MJBizDaily, April 2, 2020. https://mjbizdaily.com/states-that-have-allowed-marijuana-businesses -to-remain-open-during-coronavirus-pandemic/.

5. LeBlanc, Beth. "State Orders Owosso Barber to Close, but He's Still on the Job." The Detroit News. May 9, 2020. https://www.detroitnews.com/story/news/local/ michigan/2020/05/09/state-orders-owosso-barber-close-but-hes-still-job/3102353001/.

6. Donnelly, Francis X. "The Selling of an American Rebel: Owosso Barber Markets His Renegade Story." The Detroit News. June 15, 2020. https://www.detroit-news.com/story/news/local/michigan/2020/06/15/selling-american-rebel-owosso -barber-markets-his-story/3184472001.

7. LeBlanc, Beth Craig Munger, and Melissa Nann Burke. "High Court Strikes Down Whitmer's Emergency Powers; Gov Vows to Use Other Means." The Detroit News. October 2, 2020. https://www.detroitnews.com/story/news/local/michigan /2020/10/02/michigan-supreme-court-strikes-down-gretchen-whitmers-emergency -powers/5863340002/.

8. Associated Press. "Charges Dropped Against Barber Who Defied Whitmer, Reopened Shop." The Detroit News. October 19, 2020. https://www.detroitnews.com /story/news/local/michigan/2020/10/19/barber-defied-lockdown-reopened-charges -dropped/114444644/.

9. LeBlanc, Beth. "Owosso Barber Set to Appeal $9,000 Fine for Defying COVID Order in Court." The Detroit News. March 29, 2021. https://www.detroit-news.com/story/news/local/michigan/2021/03/29/owosso-barber-state-covid-orders -ends-saga-9000-fine/7044120002/.

10. LeBlanc, *Owosso Barber*.

11. Fauci, Anthony. "Dr. Anthony Fauci Talks With Dr. Jon LaPook About COVID-19." 60 Minutes. March 8, 2020. https://www.cbsnews.com/news/preventing -coronavirus-facemask-60-minutes-2020-03-08/.

12. Rahal, Sarah. "Amazon Workers Stage Walkout at Romulus Warehouse During COVID-19 Crisis." The Detroit News. April 1, 2020. https://www.detroit-news.com/story/news/local/wayne-county/2020/04/01/amazon-workers-stage-walk-out-romulus-warehouse-during-covid-19-crisis/5103152002/.

13. Nystrom, Mike. "MITA Requests Governor Deem Construction Operations Nonessential to Protect Employees." Michigan Infrastructure and Transportation Association. March 27, 2020. https://mi-ita.site-ym.com/news/498110/MITA -requests-Governor-deem-construction-operations-non-essential-to-protect-employ-ees.htm.

14. Rahal, Sarah. "Growing Discontent Among Some 'Essential' Workers During COVID-19 Crisis." The Detroit News. April 1, 2020. https://www.detroitnews.com /story/business/2020/04/01/growing-discontent-among-some-essential-workers-dur-ing-COVID-19-crisis/5105760002/.

15. Hunter, George. "Hundreds of Detroit Cops Back From COVID-19 Quarantine." The Detroit News. April 14, 2020. https://www.detroitnews.com/story

/news/local/detroit-city/2020/04/14/hundreds-detroit-copes-return-coronavirus-quar-antine/2992507001/.

16. LeDuff, Charlie. "Who is 'Essential?' The Underpaid and Underappreciated, It Turns Out." Deadline Detroit. March 25, 2020. https://www.deadlinedetroit.com/articles/24778/leduff_who_is_essential_the_underpaid_and-underappreciated_it_turns_out.

17. LeDuff, *Who is Essential?*

18. Amerson, Kimberly and Spencer B. Meredith, III. "The Future Operating Environment 2050: Chaos, Complexity and Competition." Small Wars Journal. July 31, 2016. https://smallwarsjournal.com/jrnl/art/the-future-operating-environment-2050-chaos-complexity-and-competition.

19. Gabbert, Bill. "Update on Gatlinburg Fires: Three People Killed." Wildfire Today. November 28, 2016. https://wildfiretoday.com/2016/11/28/wildfires-in-great-smoky-mountains-national-park-cause-evacuation. Larkin, Matt. "Gatlinburg Wildfire: Some Deaths Came From Unusual Causes, Autopsies Show." USA TODAY NETWORK – Tennessee, WFMY. August 12, 2017. https://www.9news.com/article/news/gatlinburg-wildfire-some-deaths-came-from-unusual-causes-autopsies-show/463864837.

20. Lakin, Matt. "Gatlinburg Wildfire Records Tell Story of Chaos, Confusion." Knox News. August 9, 2017. https://www.knoxnews.com/story/news/2017/08/09/gatlinburg-wildfire-records-tell-story-chaos-confusion/548412001/.

21. Kays, Holly. "Lucky to be Alive: Gatlinburg Men Relive Harrowing Escape Down Fiery Mountain." Smoky Mountain News. December 7, 2016. https://www.smokymountainnews.com/archives/item/18927-lucky-to-be-alive-gatlinburg-men-relive-harrowing-escape-down-fiery-mountain.

22. Kuligowski, Erica D., Emily H. Walpole, Ruggiero Lovreglio, and Sarah McCaffrey. "Modeling Evacuation Decision-Making in the 2016 Chimney Tops 2 Fire in Gatlinburg, TN." International Journal of Wildland Fire. September 2, 2020. DOI: 10.1071/WF20038.

23. Walpole, Emily. "Insights Into Behavior During Chimney Tops 2 Fire Could Improve Evacuation Planning." National Institute of Standards and Technology. September 2, 2020. https://www.nist.gov/news-events/news/2020/09/insights-behavior-during-chimney-tops-2-fire-could-improve-evacuation.

24. Walpole, *Insights Into Behavior.*

25. Buie, Jordan. "Franklin Resident Shares Harrowing Escape From Gatlinburg Fire." The Tennessean. December 5, 2016. https://tennessean.com/story/news/local/williamson/2016/12/05/franklin-resident-shares-harrowing-escape-gatlinburg-fire/94837496/.

26. Kays, H. *Lucky to be Alive.*

27. Ibid.

28. To protect the confidentiality of the healthcare provider and her family, she will be referred to as "Olivia," and appear as "Anonymous, Olivia" in the endnotes of this section.

29. Anonymous, Olivia, interview with the author, January 2021.

30. Time dilation. (n.d.) In *Merriam-Webster's Collegiate Dictionary.* https://www.merriam-webster.com/dictionary/time%20dilation.

31. Ghose, Tia. "Hurricane Season: How Long It Lasts and What to Expect." Live Science. December 2020. https://www.livescience.com/57671-hurricane-season .html#:~text=Savannah%2C%20Georgia%3A%20Every%201.91%20years,hit%2 075%20times%20since%201871.

32. Environmental Systems Research Institute. "Public Safety and Homeland Security Situational Awareness." ESRI White Paper. (2008): 1. http://www.esri.com /library/whitepapers/pdfs/situational-awareness.pdf.

33. Joe Dolio, interview with the author, January 31, 2021.

34. Gilbert, Sam J. "Strategic Use of Reminders: Influence of Both Domain-General and Task-Specific Metacognitive Confidence, Independent of Objective Memory Ability." *Consciousness and Cognition* 33 (2015): 245–260. 10.1016/j. concog.2015.01.006. Risko, Evan F. and Timothy L. Dunn. "Storing Information In-the-World: Metacognition and Cognitive Offloading in a Short-term Memory Task." *Consciousness and Cognition* 36 (2015): 61–74. doi: 10.1016/J. CONCOG.2015.05.014.

35. Carvalho, Jonata Tyska and Stefano Nolfi. "Cognitive Offloading Does Not Prevent but Rather Promotes Cognitive Development." *PLOS ONE* 11, no. 8 (August 2016): 3. doi: 10.1371/journal.pone.0160679.

36. Bacchi, Umberto. "Left in the Dark: Millions Hit by Internet Shutdowns in 2020." Thomson Reuters Foundation News. March 3, 2021. https://news.trust.org/ item/20210303140415-x16mh/.

37. Taye, Berhan. "Shattered Dreams and Lost Opportunities: A Year in the Fight to KeepItOn." Access Now. March 2021. https://accessnow.org/cms/assets/uploads /2021/03/KeepItOn-report-on-the-2020-data_Mar-2021_3.pdf.

38. Storm, Benjamin C., Sean M. Stone, and Aaron S. Benjamin. "Using the Internet to Access Information Inflates Future Use of the Internet to Access Other Information." *Memory* 25, no. 6. (July 18, 2016): 717–723. doi:10.1080/09658211.2 016.1210171.

39. Doug Tallman, interview with the author, May 13, 2017.

40. National Safety Council. "Preliminary Semiannual Estimates." March 4, 2021. https://injuryfacts.nsc.org/motor-vehicle/overview/preliminary-estimates/.

41. Fagnant, Daniel J. and Kara Kockleman. "Preparing a Nation for Autonomous Vehicles; Opportunities, Barriers and Policy Recommendations." *Transportation Research Part A: Policy and Practice* 77 (July 2015): 167–181.

42. Fagnant and Kockleman, *Preparing a Nation*, 167–181.

43. Stone, Linda. "Beyond Simple Multi-Tasking: Continuous Partial Attention." LindaStone.net. November 30, 2009. https://lindastone.net/2009/11/30/beyond-sim-ple-multi-tasking-continuous-partial-attention/.

44. Stone, n.d. *Homepage.* LindaStone.net.

45. Stone, n.d. *Homepage.*

46. Linda Stone, interview with the author, March 1, 2021.

47. Usborne, Simon. "The Expert Whose Children Gatecrashed His TV Interview: 'I Thought I'd Blown It in Front of the Whole World.'" The Guardian. December 20, 2017. https://www.theguardian.com/media/2017/dec/20/robert-kelly-south-korea -bbc-kids-gatecrash-viral-storm.

48. Usborne, S. *The Expert Whose Children Gatecrashed His TV Interview.*

49. Linda Stone, *Beyond Simple Multi-Tasking.*

50. Ibid.

51. Ibid.

52. Linda Stone, interview with the author, August 14, 2020.

53. Linda Stone, interview with the author, August 14, 2020.

54. Locke, Taylor. "How to Deal With Productivity-related Anxiety During the COVID-19 Pandemic, According to Experts." CNBC. March 23, 2020. https://www.cnbc.com/2020/03/23/how-to-deal-with-productivity-related-anxiety-during-covid-19.html.

55. Linda Stone, interview with the author, August 14, 2020.

56. Ibid.

57. Ibid.

58. Ibid.

59. Bose, Emily. "How to Avoid Turning Your Team Into Zoombies: The Basics." LinkedIn. May 5, 2020. https://www.linkedin.com/pulse/how-avoid-turning-your-team-zoombies-basics-emily-lewin/.

60. Linda Stone, interview with the author, August 14, 2020.

61. VanDerWerff, Emily. "How to Bake Bread: On the Existential Comforts of Coaxing Yeast Out of Air, Kneading, Proofing, Baking, and Sharing." Vox. May 19, 2020. https://www.vox.com/the-highlight/2020/5/19/21221008/how-to-bake-bread-pandemic-yeast-flour-baking-kin-forkish-claire-saffitz.

62. McKahn, Chris. "GME Stock Options Trading Explained: The Leverage Of Long Calls Against The Volatility of Game Stop." Investor's Business Daily. February 1, 2021. https://www.investors.com/research/options/gme-stock-options-buyers-got-rich-now-looking-puts/.

63. Stone, *Homepage.*

64. Lafargue, Ellen Pfeffer and Carolyn Ginsburg Stern. "Sound Solutions For A Muffled World." The ASHA Leader. American Speech-Language Hearing Association (March 2021): 54–55.

65. Lafargue and Stern, *Sound Solutions,* 54–55.

66. Amerson and Meredith, *The Future Operating Environment 2050.*

67. Juan Browne, interview with the author, January 14, 2021.

Chapter 2

Face Validity

Face validity is simple and subjective. It is a superficial assessment of whether something *appears* to make sense. A thermometer that reads 80 degrees in the middle of a snowstorm violates face validity. It is obviously broken.

Thus, face validity is about appearance. Think of an annual checkup with your doctor when you are healthy. The moment the doctor walks into the examination room, she starts to assess your presentation—body proportions, wrinkles, hygiene, posture, loudness of your greeting. Do you *appear* healthy?

Now imagine another checkup, but this time when the doctor enters the room, you are hunched over, wincing in pain, sweaty, foul-smelling, and your voice crackles. Even if you profess that you are fine, you *appear* to be ill.

And this is where face validity, which is peripheral but not inconsequential, steps aside and the concerned physician measures your vitals, listens to your respirations, and snaps the oximeter on your finger as she questions you about pain, fatigue, appetite, what you have done the past few days, and if you have been in close contact with sick people.

Next up, a blood draw and X-rays. To identify your condition and its causal factors, the doctor delves into measurements of construct, content, or criterion validity. The results of diagnostic testing then guide the doctor's approach to treatment.

In spite of its limitations, face validity often points you in the correct direction at the onset of a situation that is about to go sideways. You can efficiently recognize the incongruencies by checking normalcy bias and through thoughtful, self-aware use of your attention.

In the following sections, we will learn about face validity from a professional cyclist, a former prison inmate, and a private pilot who each perceived indicators relative to impending or unfolding crises.

THE RACE FOR INFORMATION:
NIKOLAI RAZOUVAEV[1]

On Saturday April 26, 1986, a series of procedural errors by the Chernobyl nuclear power station's staff caused one of the reactors to explode. The explosion instantly killed two employees. Another 134, including firemen, died within days and months from radiation poisoning. For the next thirty-six hours, Russian authorities suspended *Glasnost* and returned to the tried and tested omerta policy.

It did not work.

As the sun rose over the nearby town of Pripyat, residents woke up with headaches, vomiting, and a metallic taste in their mouths. Hundreds of miles away in Sweden, high radiation levels triggered an alarm at the Forsmark nuclear power plant. Concerned, the Swedes phoned Moscow only to hear the Kremlin denying any knowledge of why radiation alarms went off in Sweden.

Next morning, April 27, realizing they are dealing with an unprecedented nuclear accident, authorities evacuate Pripyat and send hundreds of buses to shuttle the residents away from the radioactive volcano.

It is at this point the gatekeepers lost control of the information they tried to conceal. When you uproot 53,000 people in one fell swoop and disperse them to villages not too far away from home without telling anyone why, rumors snowball and travel in all directions. Fast.

As misinformed people do, they mix truth with fiction, passing it from one mouth to another. No one knows what exactly is going on. By 9:00 p.m. on April 28, the unofficial official voice of the Kremlin, *Programma Vremya*, went on the air with a seventeen-second report about Chernobyl's accident. You can pack a lot into seventeen seconds, or you can tick a box and move on to the next item on the what's-truth-today menu. The news anchor ticked the box and moved on, and so did the viewers.

Thirty-six hours in, the dead, the hospitalized, the evacuated, and a handful of bureaucrats were the only ones on earth who knew what happened and, more importantly, what continued to escalate in Chernobyl. Outside of that circle, life went on as it did before April 26.

Next morning, April 29, a flight from Tashkent landed in Kiev with the Titan cycling team on board. After a stage race around Uzbekistan's capital, the team had flown to Kiev, its hometown, for a Peace Race rehearsal—a series of races organized as a drill for the upcoming Peace Race due to start from Kiev in early May.

They loaded into a team bus and headed to Prolisok, a resort on the outskirts of Kiev.

Nikolai Razouvaev, a twenty-year-old Titan rider, took the front seat across the aisle from the driver to chit chat and laugh at his latest dad jokes

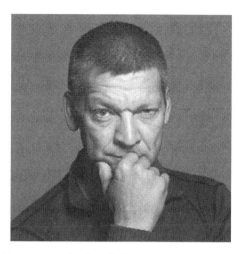

Figure 2.1 Nikolai Razouvaev. *Credit Nikolai Razouvaev.*

(figure 2.1). In a by-the-way fashion, the driver asked Nikolai if he had heard the news about the Chernobyl nuclear power plant. A North Caucasus native, unfamiliar with Ukrainian small towns' locations, Nikolai said no and asked where Chernobyl is.

For the rest of the journey, the driver shared the rumors of a nuclear disaster, told the team about evacuated Pripyat, and to stamp the rumors' authority, mentioned the *Programma Vremya* broadcast from last night. Only 100 kilometers from Kiev, he added, the nuclear plant is only 100 kilometers away as the crow flies.

At first, the extent of the news did not register in Nikolai's mind. He knew about radiation from compulsory military education classes he took in school where he had learned about nuclear weapons and their impact on life.

But this was not a nuclear attack; no one had dropped a bomb on Chernobyl. Nothing to worry about. If it were dangerous, they would have evacuated Kiev by now, all its two million residents.

He went on a training ride with the team the next morning. It was a medium tempo, two-abreast ride and he spent most of it talking with his teammate about Chernobyl. They shared the rumors and thoughts on what impact possible exposure to radiation might have on their health. Not knowing exactly what happened and the fact that Kiev continued its life as before, they agreed the rumors had probably inflated the severity of the incident.

That night, Nikolai pulled out his Selga transistor radio hoping to tune in to *Radio Svoboda* (Radio Liberty), the CIA-funded radio station established after World War II to controvert Soviet government propaganda. He had learned about *Radio Liberty* the same way he had learned about Aleksandr Solzhenitsyn—someone, he did not remember who or when, mentioned it as a piece of information you are not supposed to know. And because you are not supposed to know, you go out of your way to find out what it is.

He used to listen to *Radio Liberty* late at night, hearing stories of Soviet dissidents, political prisoners, defectors, and Kremlin insiders' shenanigans. The KGB jammed *Radio Liberty*'s Russian-language broadcasts, especially in prime time.

Everyone in the Soviet Union who ever tried to listen to *Radio Liberty* or *Voice of America* knew the jamming usually softened after midnight when authorities assumed people had already gone to bed. The government spent enormous amounts of money on radio jamming. Jamming the radio twenty-four hours a day was both expensive and impractical.

It did not take long for Nikolai to find the familiar, flat voice of a news-caster. He was talking about killed firefighters, radiation poisoning, and out of control fires still raging at the Chernobyl power plant. If true, it did not make sense to Nikolai why life in Kiev went on business as usual while a nuclear power plant was fuming radiation into the air only 100 kilometers away from Ukraine's capital.

Is it possible, if *Radio Liberty* told the truth, that the Soviet government had no problem to gamble away millions of lives because of what? Because they think they can fix the problem without telling anyone what happened?

Question was—Who do you trust? Do you trust a foreign radio station with, no doubt, its own political agenda or do you trust your eyes and act on the assumption that the government will not risk exposing millions of people to what could be a lethal dose of radiation even if the consequences of it are not immediate?

On May 1, two new indicators puzzled Nikolai even more.

The May Day parade went ahead in Kiev like it had for decades before with the entire city out on the streets celebrating the International Workers' Day. The same night, *Radio Liberty* informed its Soviet listeners that the wind in the Kiev region had changed direction from eastern to northern. It was now blowing from Chernobyl toward Kiev. If Western journalists knew this, the authorities in the Soviet Union knew this, too, but had done nothing so far.

Who do you trust?

The races Nikolai and his team came to participate in went ahead as planned. One of them, a road race on Kiev's streets, was rained on from start to finish. Nikolai remembers the jokes guys were cracking on the start line about how they would glow tomorrow from the radioactive rain and their sex lives ending next week.

No one in the peloton took the Chernobyl disaster seriously. Why would they? Not counting the rumors, no one knew what was going on. As to the rumors, there are always rumors around. And what choice did these professional racers have anyway? Pack up and go? They would fire anyone who dared to leave before they were allowed to go home.

About the same time, a new rumor, in the form of health advice, started to circulate in Kiev. Nikolai heard about red wine's unique anti-radiation properties. People said red wine shields you from the effects of radiation. *How many excuses does a Soviet male need to have a drink?* So, the guys drank, and the coaches who would otherwise fire a Titan rider if they smelled alcohol on him closed their eyes to these now-allowed antics.

Slowly, the gravity of the situation sunk into people's minds. No one thought of it as a life-or-death kind of situation, but nonetheless, death was in the air, and they did not like how it smelled. Everyone drank more red wine, just in case. More events followed and the pieces of the Chernobyl puzzle started to fall into place for Nikolai as he observed them.

He heard of people leaving Kiev in droves. Friends, and friends of friends, getting out of the city in all directions as far away from Chernobyl as possible. Driving through Kiev to Prolisok in a team car one day, he saw water trucks with cannons all over the city washing the streets and lower parts of buildings, and he recalled what he learned in those military education classes at school—running water washes away radioactive contamination.

Do you trust your eyes (face validity) or the official silence about what the eyes (and common sense) suggest is happening?

It clicked for Nikolai on one of the training rides. He saw a caravan of buses parked on the side of the road. It took a couple of minutes to pass them. At a speed of 30 km/h, the convoy must have been at least a kilometer long. One hundred of them? He didn't count. Many had what looked like lead shields bolted to the windows. None of them had the engines running. They stood on the road shoulder in cemetery silence.

As they left the buses behind, a teammate said the government wants to evacuate children from Kiev. All children. They are more vulnerable to radiation, apparently. This is what the buses are for, waiting for kids to ship them away from Kiev to save them.

It finally clicked. The picture came into focus. Chernobyl is not Hiroshima, but the radioactive poison is everywhere. How much and how bad it is still unknown, but it is clear now the rulers believe they have to start saving lives because if they do not, people will start dying.

On May 6, ten days after the reactor blew up, the Communist Party's newspaper, ironically named *Pravda* (truth), changed the gears back to *Glasnost* and published a detailed report about Chernobyl.

Two days later, the Peace Race started in Kiev as scheduled, except the Western teams refused to leave the airport when they landed, asked for a chartered plane, and when one was provided, left the USSR. The Eastern Bloc teams were ordered to stay and race every stage in Kiev as planned.

Nikolai left the Soviet Union in 1991 never to return. He lives in Australia now. Thirty-five years later, he is a healthy man, still rides, and even races his bike. One of his teammates died from cancer before reaching the age of thirty. His coach died from cancer before reaching the age of fifty. Nikolai and his former teammates do not know if these deaths were caused by the Chernobyl nuclear accident.

Face Validity in the Absence of Truth-Telling: Nikolai's Lessons

- **Actions speak louder than words.** Observe what is happening around you (situational awareness). Buses lining roads and municipal workers scrubbing down streets were signs of a government response before the nuclear accident had been acknowledged by state media.
- **Seek sources outside your area.** A transistor radio enabled Nikolai access to distal media voices not reading from the state script. Known as triangulation, the practice of using multiple sources of data or multiple perspectives enabled Nikolai to increase trustworthiness of the conclusion.
- **Share the story, not the headline.** Be patient in gathering information. Headlines focus on an important part of a story; they do not tell all. Do not be satisfied with the summaries others write. Read the stories yourself, always probing the biases and conclusions of what is written.

NO BARS BEHIND BARS: LARRY LAWTON

"How often do you really look at a man's shoes?"

In the film, *The Shawshank Redemption*, Morgan Freeman's narration of that question is juxtaposed with Tim Robbins's character walking the prison yard in the dull, dingy garb one would expect from someone behind bars—except for the shiny, polished wingtip shoes he would wear to the bank the next morning, after his escape.[2]

The popular movie line was meant to show how little attention we pay one another, but in reality, footwear offers vital information in a prison environment. So says Larry Lawton, a jewel thief turned-federal inmate turned-YouTuber and motivational speaker.

Footwear in prison was a powerful indicator of trouble, Lawton said during a June 2020 appearance on *The Safety Doc Podcast*. Especially when people deviated from normal routines. "If you saw someone with their sneakers or boots on who would normally be wearing flip flops, something's up. Something's wrong," Lawton said.[3]

It was not Lawton's muscular frame that kept him safe in prison, he said, but rather a keen awareness of when trouble was afoot. "Is something about to go down? Is someone going to be stabbed? Is there going to be a riot? Are two gangs going to go at it?" Lawton said, sharing some of the questions he asked himself after seeing warning signs.[4]

After spending 1996 to 2007 behind bars, Lawton was immortalized as a character in the video game *Grand Theft Auto 5*, became a YouTuber with 1.5 million subscribers, and offers coaching and motivational speeches to troubled youth.

9/11 behind Bars: A Test of Face Validity

Before his 1996 arrest and 1997 guilty plea, Lawton stole some fifteen million dollars' worth of jewels up and down the East Coast.[5] Lawton was in federal prison in Jessup, Georgia during the September 11 terror attacks. He was in his cell reading a book when the first plane hit the World Trade Center.

A fellow inmate, hailing from Lawton's native New York, had been watching one of the TVs in the common area. He alerted Lawton, "Larry, a plane just hit the World Trade Center," his friend said.

Hearing the news before seeing it, Lawton first thought the plane was more like a Cessna, a personal aircraft. And not the Boeing 767 that did crash.

He got to the TV room in time to see the second plane hit. He and the other inmates spent the day as many Americans did: watching TV, trying to make sense of it all. Unlike most Americans, they were unable to change the channel.

But in the wake of the terror attacks, when the Federal Bureau of Prisons system went on a lockdown, that is when the flow of information really slowed. "That hurt us worse," Lawton said. "Now we're locked in our cells, not knowing what's going on." No one had a TV in their cell in federal prison, but some people, including Lawton, did have transistor radios. Those radios became their lifeline to the news of the world and offered more choice than the one channel of TV news they relied on before.

Lawton said that "after about a week, then some crazy shit started coming in," as inmates took what little information they had and added more onto it, including conspiracy theories about who "really" carried out the attacks. In the absence of reliable information, heard by everyone watching the same TV at the same time, the prisoners played their own game of Telephone.

In the game of Telephone, kids sit in a circle. One child whispers a message to the next—for example, "A baby shark swims in the ocean"—who whispers it to the next, and so on. The object is for the message to stay the same, from the first kid to the last. The object lesson is that it is human nature to add on something extra. Somewhere on that telephone line, someone always decides to add or omit a word, or to change the phrase entirely.

Playing Telephone is a one-way act of faith where one can parrot what they have been told, but cannot be sure they were told the correct original message. Telephone would be a dangerous game in prison where the face validity of any new information is low, as everyone in the building benefits from manipulating whoever they can, however they can.

Bad information can walk someone into danger. But asking questions is rarely the safe move, and at any rate would generally yield unreliable information. "You have to read between the lines," Lawton said.

In a prison environment, the line between friend and foe is blurry and smudged often. Safety in prison demands assessing what you are being told, the messenger, and what motivations that person might have all without appearing to be doing so.

Think for Yourself: The Value of Debate

"I feel bad for very vulnerable young people, who haven't been around in life enough to realize what they should really listen to and what they shouldn't," Lawton said.[6] He wrote a book about his experiences called *Gangster Redemption* and mentors young people to avoid the mistakes that result in prison time.

Lawton urges people to use their own judgment on what works and what does not. His goal is not to give them the answers, but to help them ask the right questions as they navigate a world that rarely has their best interests at heart. "Filter the good stuff, and throw out the stuff you don't want," Lawton said.[7]

Debate has been a useful tool, Lawton said, in helping young people build critical thinking skills. He will choose an issue and assign kids to argue in favor or against. "But I don't like the issue," kids will often complain. That is when Lawton gets to explain the real purpose of the exercise.

Debate is not about getting kids to say what they do not believe; it is about getting them to understand the soundness and weakness of arguments, regardless of what they believe. "Then they get more information, and they start looking at things differently," Lawton said. "That's how I help young people decipher information from one source to another."[8]

Back to the Wall

Lawton said that when he meets a friend in law enforcement at a restaurant, they will both try to be seated against the wall, facing the door, with a line of sight on who is coming and who is going. When see they are going for the same spot, they will laugh. "I want to make sure my blind side is covered," Lawton said.[9]

For Lawton, vigilance is the gift that his time in prison keeps on giving. Corrections officers, who spend nearly as much time behind bars as prisoners, often experience "hypervigilance" as a carryover from their work lives to home.

Where they sit at restaurants or movie theaters is shaped by their heightened perception of risk. That perception of risk owes to regular exposure to violence at work. Even when they are off duty, they see threat potential, those indicators, everywhere. Lawton, twelve years an inmate, does too.

A person whose back is against the wall cannot be stabbed in the back—they would at least see the attack coming and be in a better position to react. In prison, situational awareness was a matter of life and death, Lawton said. Inmates who walked around unaware were called "out to lunch" or "tourists" at risk of attack and not even knowing it.

Beyond the prison walls, Lawton said, the thought is not so much about personal security anymore, but being able to see and stop a danger to the public before things turn grave. "I want to be there so I can prevent something from happening," Lawton said.

Lawton's Lessons: Face Validity in a Masked World

- **Read between the lines.** Take nothing at face value. Is the information fact, or opinion? Or both? Is it offered to inform, or to advocate? What does the author want me to think? Who benefits from me thinking that way?
- **Consider the source, and their motivations.** On Lawton's transistor radio, some hosts would be leftists and others would be right-wing. Truth was sifted by comparing information from those sources with that from other prisoners, with contacts from the outside world, and with corrections officers, who have a foot in both camps.
- **Information is a giant buffet line.** Truth is found in the weighing and measuring of multiple sources of information. Sole reliance on any one source raises the odds of giving credence to misinformation. Take what is useful, and to taste, and leave the rest for others.

JUAN BROWNE, THE OROVILLE DAM, AND THE CITIZEN-AS-JOURNALIST

Juan Browne did not set out to be a citizen journalist when he took to the sky to investigate the buzz about the service, or primary, spillway failure at the Oroville Dam, upstream of Sacramento in Northern California. He was simply curious. And in a time crunch. "I had this little airplane, and I just flew over there out of curiosity," Browne said in a January 2021 interview. "I just wanted to see what was going on."[10]

A spillway conveys water past a dam and is necessary for regulating the capacity of the reservoir. With its suddenly disintegrating concrete chute, the Oroville service spillway was no longer able to operate as engineered—and the reservoir water level was rising.

On February 11, 2017, Oroville Dam, America's tallest, at 770 feet, overtopped and damaged its emergency spillway for the first time in its history, forcing the evacuation of nearly 200,000 people.[11] The unnatural disaster took about one billion dollars to repair and caused millions more in property damage (figure 2.2).[12]

Just one day prior to the incident, on February 10, Browne made his first video about the dam. Fearing that the government would soon restrict air traffic over the site, Browne, a commercial pilot for American Airlines, got

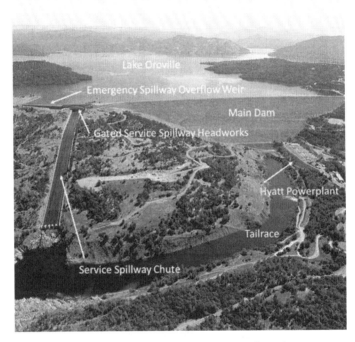

Figure 2.2 Overview of Oroville Dam Facility Prior to the February 2017 Incident. *Credit Irfan Alvi;* The Oroville Dam image was originally published in the Independent Forensic Team Report Oroville Dam Spillway Incident as Figure 3-1 on January 5, 2018. On August 28, 2021, Irfan A. Alvi granted the author permission to use the figure in this book.

into his 1946 Luscombe 8A single-engine plane to offer the world the rarest of bird's-eye view.

Browne used a GoPro Hero5 camera to shoot the video. He added narration and published it to his YouTube channel, @blancolirio, the next day. The video immediately went viral. It has since amassed more than 500,000 views.[13]

In the five-minute, ten-second video, Browne shows a command of the scene, the situation, and the possible consequences of the dam's failure.[14] The view from 3,000 feet is intimate and dramatic. With no other planes in the sky, and no people at the site, the rarity of the vantage is apparent. One gets the feeling of being led on a backstage tour.

Throughout, Browne's tone is even and informative, never breathless or excited. "That's the big concern going forward: how much erosion are we going to get?" Browne says at one point, summarizing the fears of his neighbors who were watching.[15] That concern was justified.

Costing in excess of one billion dollars, the repair effort required months of around-the-clock effort by 600 staffers and contractors of the California Department of Water Resources and Kiewit Infrastructure.[16] "I realized right away that we hit a nerve here," Browne said in a January 2021 interview. "A lot of people had a lot of good questions about it. And I felt obligated to continue to answer them."[17]

He began to make more videos.

The Message Makes the Medium

A YouTube star was born. But it took more than six years for Browne's channel, @blancolirio, to become an overnight success. It was not the medium that explained Browne's newfound reach or his now-massive fan base of 300,000 subscribers. It was the message.

Browne had been a YouTuber for more than a half-decade before the Oroville Dam video. He would upload videos from the town's Mardi Gras parade or from a motorcycle ride, or from around the house, and get a few hundred views. Up in the air, seeking truth, and answering the questions that mattered to neighbors fearing for their futures is when things took off for his channel.

"Just the Facts:" Privilege and Unfair Advantages

Obviously, not everyone has the means to earn a pilot license or to own a hobby plane. But those resources do not tell the story of Juan Browne's success as a citizen journalist, not any more than his YouTube account does.

Browne has been a licensed pilot since age sixteen. He has been flying longer than he has been driving. If a plane and a GoPro and a YouTube account were all it took to go viral, Juan Browne would have done it before February 2017. The story of Juan Browne is not that of a privileged man who owned a plane, but that of a citizen who leveraged his privilege to deliver the information others could not.

As the months-long repair effort went on, Browne continued his reports. Over time, he was perceived as an honest broker by the state and the engineering firm, and was allowed a unique level of access to the dam (figure 2.3). "Nobody else was really doing it with this level of detail or interest," Browne said.[18]

That August, six months after the failure, Browne allowed a newspaper reporter to tag along on a tour of the dam site. "As he introduced himself to workers with the Department of Water Resources and Kiewit Infrastructure Company, he was met with nods of both acknowledgement and approval once they realized he was the guy producing all those videos," *The Union* newspaper reported.[19] "'This guy gets it,' was heard more than once with all the handshakes," the story read.[20]

Browne's work as a hobbyist is why the professional news reporter was allowed to take the tour. For most of American history, it would have been the other way around. In this information age, status is not conferred by job titles, but by work product. If it was the plane that offered Browne a vantage others did not have in that first video, it was his curious approach that allowed for everything else.

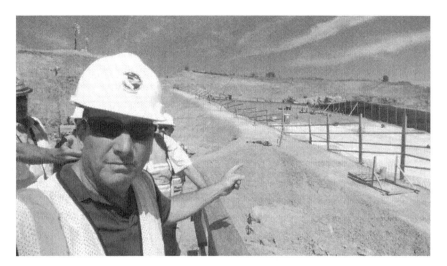

Figure 2.3   Juan Browne observes repairs to the Oroville service spillway – credit Juan Browne.

Indeed, *not* having a media badge allowed workers at the site to share information more freely with Browne than they might have otherwise if they feared a bad or an out-of-context quote would be blown up into a front-page headline. "Every time a mainstream news person would come in there, they would immediately put some kind of spin on this thing," Browne said.[21]

The lesson of Juan Browne is not to get a plane, but to develop a nose for new information, and a teacher's interest in sharing it. Browne said his video reports were motivated, in part, by a lack of unspun, unslanted information from the news media.

He also believes that is why the public responded so strongly. "There is a huge void, or a huge market for, just the facts," Browne said.[22] "People really responded to that, and it seems to be so lacking in today's modern infotainment industry. They just wanted the facts."[23]

Years later, the Oroville Dam situation is history, no longer current events. But the pivot brought on by that February 2017 report continues. After Kobe Bryant's fatal January 2020 helicopter crash, Browne leveraged his background as a pilot to help the public understand the factors leading up to it, and the government reports issued on the crash.

And in May 2020, after the Midland Dam collapse in Michigan, Browne leveraged his background with historic dam bursts to offer another video explaining the newest one.[24] This time, he did not need to live a half-hour away or to fly a plane over it to explain things.

So valued is Browne's knowledge of dam failures that his Midland Dam video has 300,000 more views than the original Oroville Dam video.

Lessons in Citizen Journalism from Juan Browne

- **See it for yourself.** The news does not come to you unspun or unslanted. If you really want to know, go. This effort does not require a plane in most cases. But the answers you want will not come find you. You have to go find them.
- **You have not because you ask not.** Ask questions. Asking questions does not require a media badge, and sometimes you can get better answers without one. Identify who has the answers to your questions and ask them.
- **Be curious, not cunning.** Excuse people for their personal foibles and be non-judgmental about official failures. It is information you want, not "gotcha" headlines.

The rise of the citizen-as-journalist both coincides with, and is a reaction to, the general public's desire to eliminate perceived or real bias in their news reporting. It is a trend that is likely to continue as long as bias exists.

BIASES

A bias is an inclination—either consciously realized or completely unknown to a person (or group)—to present or be predisposed toward a particular perspective. How we perceive information is strongly influenced by our past experiences. An analytical stumbling block of human thinking is the expectation of a future that is similar to the past.

The unconscious desire to remain in our comfortable torus is powerful and contributes greatly to cognitive bias in any given situation. The following chapters discuss common cognitive biases. Consider how some or all of these biases appeared in the stories shared by Nikolai Razouvaev, Larry Lawton, and Juan Browne (figure 2.4).

The Supply Chain Is Breaking: Expectations and Default Bias

On April 26, 2020, Tyson Foods took out a full-page ad in *The New York Times*. "As pork, beef and chicken plants are being forced to close, even for short periods of time, millions of pounds of meat will disappear from the supply chain," stated John Tyson, chairman of Tyson Foods.[25] He added, "As a result, there will be limited supply of our products available in grocery stores until we are able to reopen our facilities that are currently closed."[26]

Tyson's advertisement was hyperbole and focused hungry American eyes on Congress to feed stimulus dollars to corporations. The supply chain was under tension, but Tyson's decree of a fragile supply chain was incomplete. It would twist, bend, and groan, but it was not going to fracture. Tyson was counting on the exploitation of different biases in American consumers.

First, we know that supply networks in America have proven resilient for short-term, regionalized chaos events such as hurricanes. Transportation and logistics management have come a long way in the past decade.

Conditioned by fear from constant reports regarding the severity of the COVID-19 pandemic, Americans were expecting negative news (expectations bias). Tyson's message was thus delivered on point.

Next, supply systems have become highly efficient over the past thirty years and have consequently driven down costs for items. By the 1990s, "Just in Time" manufacturing (JIT) was being adopted across industries—including productions of firearms and ammunition. How did we get here?

JIT manufacturing has its origins to the 1970s Toyota plants in Japan. The purpose of JIT is to limit warehousing of items and instead have items manufactured and sent directly to suppliers and to customers. This method is especially prominent in modern book publishing where the book is not printed until the customer places an order. Instead of retrieving a copy from

Perceptual Biases	Biases in Evaluating Evidence
Expectations. We tend to perceive what we expect to perceive. More (unambiguous) information is needed to recognize an unexpected phenomenon.	**Consistency.** Conclusions drawn from a small body of consistent data engender more confidence than ones drawn from a larger body of less consistent data.
Resistance. Perceptions resist change even in the face of new evidence.	**Missing Information.** It is difficult to judge well the potential impact of missing evidence, even if the information gap is known.
Ambiguities. Initial exposure to ambiguous or blurred stimuli interferes with accurate perception, even after more and better information becomes available.	**Discredited Evidence.** Even though evidence supporting a perception may be proved wrong, the perception may not quickly change.
Biases in Estimating Probabilities	Biases in Perceiving Causality
Availability. Probability estimates are influenced by how easily one can imagine an event or recall similar instances.	**Rationality.** Events are seen as part of an orderly, causal pattern. Randomness, accident, and error tend to be rejected as explanations for observed events.
Anchoring. Probability estimates are adjusted only incrementally in response to new information or further analysis.	**Attribution.** Behavior of others is attributed to some fixed nature of the person or country, while our own behavior is attributed to the situation in which we find ourselves.
Overconfidence. In translating feelings of certainty into a probability estimate, people are often overconfident, especially if they have considerable expertise.	**Jumping to Conclusions.** The tendency to stop collecting evidence sooner than others and then make decisions based on limited, or irrelevant, contextual information.

Figure 2.4 Common Perceptual and Cognitive Biases. *Credit United States Central Intelligence Agency;* United States. Central Intelligence Agency. "A Tradecraft Primer: Structured Analytic Techniques for Improving Intelligence Analysis." Central Intelligence Agency. March 2009 [modified April 28, 2009; cited May 5, 2017.] Adapted from Figure-Common Perceptual and Cognitive Biases: 6. https://www.hsdl.org/?abstract&did=20945.

a pallet in a warehouse, the book is printed after it is ordered and then is sent directly to the buyer.

Tyson, along with all manufacturers, has benefited greatly from JIT, but there is a notable disadvantage to JIT in the midst of prolonged, or national, chaos. There is no spare finished product available to meet unexpected orders, because all products are made to meet actual orders. When demand skyrockets, as it has for popular types of rifle ammunition in 2020, production can only scale up so much and backorders extend for months or even years.[27]

When a chaos event is severe or prolonged, agreements crumble as was seen in the disruptions of raw materials for common kinds of plastics:

> This [the COVID-19 lockdowns and effects of Hurricane Laura] was followed by a slew of force majeures from big polymer producers, including LyondellBasell in Louisiana and Chevron Phillips Chemical in Texas. (By declaring force majeure, these suppliers were relieved of certain supply-delivery commitments due to circumstances outside their control.) Simultaneously, Covid-19 safety precautions slowed production at many workplaces and caused labor and trucking shortages at ports.[28]

JIT is not the endgame because raw materials must be sourced and transported. Whatever polymers, pellets, and dyes we load into our 3D printers do not come from backyard mining.

Nevertheless, the plummeting costs of 3D printers (also referred to as additive manufacturing) already enable the average household to skip the store and print their own stands for smartphones or articulated robot toys for children.

3D printing is also having a revolutionary effect on manufacturing. For example, with traditional manufacturing processes, each new part or change in part design requires a new tool, mold, dye, or jig to be manufactured to create the new part. In 3D printing, the design is fed into slicer software, needed supports added, and then it is printed with little or no change at all in the physical machinery or equipment. And drawings of files for 3D printed items are increasingly shared between the professional 3D community, social media users, and individual citizens.

Researchers studying how 3D printing and social media tackled the PPE shortage during COVID-19 found, "more than 140 Social Media Groups from 36 countries and more than 18,000 individual members participated in the 3D printing effort for Covid 19 to make printable masks, face shields, and ventilators."[29] This finding demonstrates a profound effect on real-world supply chain logistics.

> The supply chain is, in fact, shedding links. Belgian chocolate is world-renowned for its quality. Now, a factory in Belgium called Miam ("yum" in French) is using four specialty 3D printers to create ready-to-eat delectable edibles from milk chocolate, dark chocolate or white chocolate. A nearby brewery commissioned The Miam Factory to 3D print chocolate beer bottles that served as memorable awards following an Easter egg hunt.[30]

The 3D printing market is set to double in size every three years with the annual growth forecasted by analysts varying between 18.2 and 27.2 percent.[31] It will be astounding to examine a fifty-year sample of the supply chain from 1980 to 2030 and note the progression from warehousing to JIT to 3D.

Eventually, the aim is to have a 3D printer in your kitchen that creates meals for you on demand. With a simple download of a file that includes your nutritional requirements, taste profile, allergy information, etc., this printer would go on to create or print meals in a matter of minutes.[32]

Chaos is associated with danger and uncertainty. That is our default bias. We perceive a chaos event as degrading an existing social structure or mechanical system. Our focus is on immediate concerns, but we need to invest some perspective toward chaos as a catalyst for widespread, and positive, change.

Some of the most critical innovations in common use today rose out of chaotic instances in the past. The ability to mass produce antibiotics resulted from the staggering battlefield losses due to infection during World War I and previous altercations. Air travel went from a novel concept prior to World War I to the use of jet propulsion systems on every aircraft after World War II. The launch of the computer age started with code breaking mathematics machines in the 1940s that morphed into the phones we use every day. The origins of the Internet began as a way for Defense Department officials to pass along information in a fast, effective and secure way during the Cold War.[33]

Eating a 3D printed meal is only cringeworthy because so far, we only know meals that have not been 3D printed. Move from the default bias that chaos is bad until proven good. Accept that change is the only constant in life. Disruption does not set us back, but instead propels us forward.

Rightly or wrongly, expectations bias and default bias both contribute to a mental baseline we use to evaluate events and information. We also need to be aware of additional biases that color our reactions to information and information processing.

NEGATIVE VICARIOUS REHEARSAL

Stressed and anxious people are susceptible to perceptual and cognitive biases. Some demonstrate a behavior known as negative vicarious rehearsal which can skew resource allocations and priorities (such as spending more on personal defense and less on nutritious foods) and heavily tax response and recovery systems.

The communication age gives national audiences the experience of local crises. Examples include the media coverage of urban, localized riots in 2020. What people saw depended on from where they got their news—but all of the big networks were centered on the most dramatic scenes. In reality, only a small number of cities declared curfews and braced for violence. National protests about police brutality and racial justice remained largely peaceful.

The media abhors an information vacuum. It will take what information it has and amplify it, completing the ensemble with speculation when deemed necessary. Uncertainty makes us crave more information, so many people spend a lot of time looking for news updates, refreshing screens every few minutes to seek reassurance. As people lose proportion and perspective, they spiral down a whirlpool of confirmation (expectation) bias.

Because these targeted messages (such as board up your windows and stay home) were splashed across the Internet, they also reached people who did not need to take immediate action. Some unaffected observers mentally rehearsed the localized riots crisis as if they were experiencing it and practiced the courses of action presented to them. This group included rural store owners closing their businesses and stacking pallets and other items to barricade entrances.

People bought firearms. Concerned about their safety, many decided that they were at the same level of risk as those directly affected by civil unrest and they needed *the ultimate* remedy.

The week starting March 16, the FBI conducted 1.2 million background checks—the most in a single week that the FBI has on record. The highest single day on the record is March 20, with 210,308 total checks across the US. Gun stores saw empty shelves, as retailers struggled to keep up with demand.[34]

In a July 2020 interview with NPR reporter Chris Arnold, Mandy Collins of Little Mountain, South Carolina (population 291), with her husband and three kids, said she decided to purchase her first gun.[35] "With all the toilet paper gone and everything, people just started acting crazy," she says. "I guess the fear of the unknown and letting prisoners out of prison, and I just '. . .' decided I wanted to go ahead and just purchase one."[36]

While Mandy Collin's purchase might yield a heightened sense of personal safety, it did not make her safer from COVID-19 and it probably increased her attention to the media-driven dangers of rioting that were out of proportion to any real risk. It is a self-reinforcing spiral, or even panic, and a bump in the night or an unfamiliar car turning around in the driveway can make new gun owners think, "Should I reach for my firearm?"

When people's thoughts were not fixated on firing a shot in self-defense, they were still worrying about receiving a shot for immunity from COVID-19.

Early in the vaccine rollout, mainstream media eagerly featured stories of vaccine distribution challenges, although these occurrences were to be anticipated due to temporary supply shortage, clinical staffing limitations, and communication gaps in making people aware of rollout procedures.

Due to these media-stoked fears, we would again witness widespread negative vicarious rehearsal from people zig-zagging regions in search of vaccinations and rejecting the prioritized rollout of vaccinations to specific groups of people with a higher risk of COVID-19 infection. The initial spike in demand for vaccines, coupled with dire reporting in the media, caused a spiral of panic among anxious people susceptible to negative vicarious rehearsal. These reactions were often compounded by a phenomenon known as conjunction fallacy, another type of bias.

CONJUNCTION FALLACY: MR. F. HAD A HEART ATTACK

In 1983, world-renowned psychologists Amos Tversky and Daniel Kahneman published a ground-breaking study on intuitive human cognitive bias.[37] They showed that when subjects are asked the likelihood of several alternatives, including single and joint events, they often make a conjunction fallacy. That is, they rate the conjunction of two events as being more likely, or more plausible, than only one of the constituent events.

They presented the following fabricated scenarios to 115 undergraduates at Stanford University and the University of British Columbia:

A health survey was conducted in a representative sample of adult males in British Columbia of all ages and occupations. Mr. F. was included in the sample. He was selected by chance from a list of participants. Which of the following statements is more probable?

(A) Mr. F. has had one or more heart attacks.
(B) Mr. F. has had one or more heart attacks and he is over 55 years old.

This seemingly transparent problem elicited a substantial proportion (58% selected option B) of conjunction errors among statistically naive respondents.[38]

This example, and countless like it, reveal that we are all subject to the conjunction fallacy, where we regularly violate the laws of probability due to a vivid story. This error in decision-making happens when people judge that a conjunction of two possible events is more likely than one or both of the conjuncts.

Innate human reasoning infers that the addition of more details increases the probability of two events occurring simultaneously. (It is also an explanation for why liars tend to add additional or even excessive detail to a given lie in order to predispose the recipient to accepting the lie as truth.) However, the more detailed outcome is just that, more detailed. It is not more plausible or more likely.

In fact, the probability of the two events occurring together (in conjunction) is always less than or equal to the probability of either one occurring alone. In other words, a conjunction cannot be more probable than one of its constituents.

Which of these statements might you have deemed to be most probable on March 25, 2020?

(A) The governor has ordered people to stay home.
(B) The governor has ordered people to stay home, and state highways are closed.

Previous studies of conjunction statements imply that the majority of people presented with these statements would select B. Fortunately, conjunction bias collapses in on itself when too many conditions are stated. Most people are able to identify the mental trickery of a statement with a dozen conjunctions. It no longer makes sense from a face validity standpoint.

Recognizing one's own biases, such as expectations and default bias, as well as tendencies toward negative vicarious rehearsal and conjunction fallacy, goes a long way toward improving the ability to vet informational inputs correctly. In chapter 3, we will explore one solid method of eliminating biases and verifying indicators and information through implementing member check networks.

NOTES

1. Nikolai Razouvaev, personal communications with the author, January 2021 to April 2021.
2. *The Shawshank Redemption*. Directed by Frank Darabont. Mansfield, OH: Columbia Pictures, 1994. DVD.

3. Larry Lawton, "Situational Awareness in Prison." Interview by David P. Perrodin. *The Safety Doc Podcast*, June 23, 2020. https://youtu.be/d9hcg2pavVU.

4. Lawton, *Situational Awareness in Prison.*

5. Wolford, Ben. "Ex-Jewel Robber Seeks Redemption Through Mentoring." South Florida Sun Sentinel. April 14, 2013. https://www.sun-sentinel.com/news/fl -xpm-2013-04-14-fl-jewel-thief-20130405-story.html.

6. Lawton, *Situational Awareness in Prison.*

7. Ibid.

8. Ibid.

9. Ibid.

10. Juan Browne, personal communication with the author, January 14, 2021.

11. France, John W., Irfan A. Alvi, Peter A. Dickson, Henry T. Falvey, Stephen J. Rigbey, and John Trojanowski. Independent Forensic Team Report for Oroville Dam Spillway Incident. January 5, 2018: 8, 26. https://damsafety.org/sites/default/files/ files/Independent%20Forensic%20Team%20Report%20Final%2001-05-18.pdf.

12. Alvi, Irfan. "Case Study: Oroville Dam, California." Dam Failures. 2018. https://damfailures.org/case-study/oroville-dam-california-2017/.

13. Juan Browne. "Oroville Spillway Failure Flyover and Explanation." February 10, 2017. https://youtu.be/_2aD53JIDzo.

14. Juan Browne, *Oroville Spillway Failure Flyover.*

15. Ibid.

16. Hamilton, Brian. "Massive Effort in Motion to Repair Oroville Dam Spillway." The Union. August 30, 2017. https://www.theunion.com/news/local-news /massive-effort-in-motion-to-repair-oroville-dam-spillway/.

17. Juan Browne, personal communication.

18. Ibid.

19. Hamilton, *Massive Effort in Motion.*

20. Ibid.

21. Juan Browne, personal communication.

22. Ibid.

23. Ibid.

24. Juan Browne. "Michigan Dam(s) Fail! Tittabawassee River." May 20, 2020. https://youtu.be/XpZMb5TR-hU.

25. Tyson, John H. "Tyson Ad." The Washington Post. April 27, 2020. https://www .washingtonpost.com/context/tyson-ad/86b9290d-115b-4628-ad80-0e679dcd2669/ ?itid=lk_inline_manual_2.

26. Tyson, *Tyson Ad.*

27. Hoover, Matthew. "Four Waves of Chaos—Where is All the Ammunition?" Interview by David P. Perrodin. *The Safety Doc Podcast*, September 5, 2020. http:// safetyphd.com/safety-doc-livestream-148-matthew-hoover-four-waves-of-chaos -where-is-all-the-ammunition/.

28. Vakil, Bindiya. "The Latest Supply Chain Disruption: Plastics." Harvard Business Review. March 26, 2021.

29. Vordos, Nick, Despina A. Gkika, George Maliaris, Konstantinos E. Tilkeridis, Anastasia Antoniou, Dimitrios V. Bandekas, and Athanasios Ch. Mitropoulos.

"How 3D Printing and Social Media Tackles the PPE Shortage During Covid-19 Pandemic." *Safety Science* 130 (2020): 104870. doi: 10.1016/j.ssci.2020.104870.

30. GE. "How 3D-Printed Food Could Change the Way We Cook and Eat." GE Additive. 2020. https://www.ge.com/additive/additive-manufacturing/industries/food -beverage.

31. AMFG Autonomous Manufacturing. "40+ 3D Printing Industry Stats You Should Know." January 14, 2020. https://amfg.ai/2020/01/14/40-3d-printing-industry -stats-you-should-know-2020-redirect/.

32. Alexander, Donovan. "3D Printing Will Change the Way You Eat in 2020 and Beyond." Interesting Engineering. March 27, 2020. https://interestingengineering .com/3d-printing-will-change-the-way-you-eat-in-2020-and-beyond.

33. Stuart, Jordan. "Rising to the Challenge. Insights on the Innovation and Opportunities that Arise out of Difficult Times." Federated Hermes. March 30, 2020.

34. Taylor, Kate. "Gun Sales Boomed in 2020, With Background Checks Hitting Record Highs as Millions of People Bought Guns for the First Time." Business Insider. January 15, 2021. https://www.businessinsider.com/gun-sales-boom-2020 -background-checks-hit-record-highs-2021-1.

35. DataUSA. n.d. https://datausa.io/profile/geo/little-mountain-sc.

36. Arnold, Chris. "Pandemic and Protests Spark Record Gun Sales." National Public Radio. July 16, 2020. https://www.npr.org/2020/07/16/891608244/protests -and-pandemic-spark-record-gun-sales.

37. Tversky, Amos and Daniel Kahneman. "Extensional Versus Intuitive Reasoning: The Conjunction Fallacy in Probability Judgment." *Psychological Review* 90 (1983): 293–315.

38. Tversky and Kahneman, *Extensional Versus Intuitive Reasoning*, 293–315.

Chapter 3

Member Check Network

FORCE MULTIPLIERS

If you hang around someone with a military background long enough, you might end up hearing a term called "force multiplier." In a combat context, a force multiplier might simply mean more troops and weapons than the opponent. Leveraging weather, season, terrain, specialized training, and even surprise might enable a numerically inferior force to prevail in battle.

Integrated security systems can be force multipliers, such as connecting a neighborhood's doorbell cameras to create a surveillance mosaic. A drone with a camera exponentially strengthens the effectiveness of ground-based search and rescue personnel.

Assembling a group of people to observe and then report what is happening in their setting is a special form of force multiplier known as a member check network. We will read more about that later in this section.

Force multipliers make it easier to gather information, but do they simplify decision-making?

DECISION-MAKING BASICS

Simply presenting causal information to people may not help them make decisions. In their study, "How Causal Information Affects Decision," researcher Mia Zheng and her colleagues made a potent discovery:

> Simply presenting more information to people may not have the intended effects, particularly when they must combine this information with their existing knowledge and beliefs. While psychological studies have shown that causal

models can be used to choose interventions and predict outcomes, that work has not tested structures of the complexity found in machine learning, or how such information is interpreted in the context of existing knowledge.[1]

The team proposes this has something to do with our existing mental models. We do not take causal information at face value; instead, our existing beliefs and experience influence our decisions. This phenomenon can sometimes mean we do not make the right choice.

With extra information, we can lose confidence and start second-guessing ourselves. In addition to addressing internal bias and prior knowledge influencing decision-making, we must also reckon with the conundrum that is the decision-making process.

Few people are ever taught how to make a decision. It is either something a person is assumed to have learned throughout life or is taught as a sequenced process. In order to make a decision, you need to have a critical thinking process to consider information.

A well-known method to evaluate information for intelligence purposes is the Admiralty System (alternatively called the NATO system). It is a heuristic tool used to demonstrate the net worth of a particular piece of information based on both source reliability and data validity (figure 3.1).[2]

Joe Dolio, the corporate security investigator, and his member checks used the Admiralty System to sift and winnow the trove of information pouring in during 2020. During an interview, he flipped back the pages from his go-everywhere clipboard, revealing a heavily scratched, transparent plastic laminate film—beneath it, the rating criteria of the Admiralty System.

Versions of this alphanumeric grading system are used by police forces and security firms around the world. This straightforward tool, which could be inscribed on a notecard, can be used by adults and older children.

Source Reliability	*Information Credibility*
A. Completely reliable	1. Confirmed by other sources
B. Usually reliable	2. Probably true
C. Fairly reliable	3. Possibly true
D. Not usually reliable	4. Doubtful
E. Unreliable	5. Improbable
F. Reliability cannot be judged	6. Truth cannot be judged

Figure 3.1 Admiralty Scale for Source and Info Evaluation. *Credit Joseph and Corkill (also credited in endnote #3); Table 2 adapted from Joseph and Corkill, Information Evaluation, 5.*

The Admiralty Scale provides a means of discerning between the credibility of various information sources. Humans do not seem to have an innate ability to do so without building such systems.

In a study comparing information sources used by the public during two infectious disease outbreaks (SARS and H1N1), researchers found that people seldom consulted credible sources, such as their doctor, on a frequent basis.[3]

Additionally, the ubiquitous nature of information in the Internet Age means that people have more opportunities to acquire information that was previously unavailable to the public. However, it did not necessarily make them understand risks and arrive at informed decisions.[4]

"'More is better' only if the additional information sources can contribute to better informed decision-making; otherwise use of multiple sources can create confusion about agency credibility and appropriate health risk behaviours that may cause more harm than good."[5]

The researchers learned that friends and relatives were commonly used as an information source but were simultaneously not deemed very useful or credible.[6] While family and friends are often supportive during uncertain times, they are unlikely to be more knowledgeable about the situation than you are—and because of that limitation, it is important to avoid miscasting them as a bona fide member check network that is using, with fidelity, a tried-and-true tool to evaluate information. However, a member check network that is composed of people outside of family and friends can be highly effective.

When a small group of five or six people collaborate to develop a member check network, everyone is a contributor to the network. One person (or more, depending upon number of contributors in the group) serves as the primary collector (PC).

The PC is responsible for teaching contributors the Admiralty Scale to promote inter-rater reliability across contributors. The PC, who analyzes submitted data, is also in the best position to winnow cumulative information into intelligence and report that back to contributors. In some instances, summative information might be shared with people who subscribe to the network, but have no role in informing it. The PC is also tasked with curating and archiving data. A member check network is not bound to a maximum size. But there is no benefit in an organization being a mile wide and an inch deep. Ordinary citizens Charles Mak and Bryan Bowden have both found and contributed value to their member check network through active participation.

LEFT TO HIS OWN DEVICES: CHARLES MAK

Charles Mak lived in Pittsburgh during the COVID-19 pandemic.[7] He contributed to a small member check network that consisted of people living in the United States and Canada.

At three-day intervals, the members shared observations specific to their locality including: government decrees, behavior of the public, availability of food and supplies, and use of PPE by government workers, including postal carriers. Network members believed these indicators could be reliably measured by each member and might predict the proliferation of conditions, such as shortages of canned foods or the closing of schools or workplaces.

Sometimes the hill you die on is your own front porch if your bare hand grazes the COVID-19 contaminated mailbox.

The member check network agreed that observing postal carriers wearing gloves, face shields, or masks would be an indicator of elevated public risks associated with COVID-19. In other words, if postal carriers dressed like Superfund technicians or engaged in rituals of UV wand waving and disinfectant aerosol misting upon their routes, those would be signs for everyone else to prepare for a potential shutdown of not just the mail, but all home deliveries.

One member reported a postal carrier wearing gloves and a mask, but also not changing the gloves between mail deliveries to different properties.[8] The postal carriers would be, per the members, canaries in the coal mine, and through five months of scheduled check-ins, the behavior of postal carriers, out and about in communities, remained largely unchanged.[9]

The initial two weeks of pandemic preparation at Mak's medical facility centered on increasing capacity for a swell of patients and possibly housing staff in nearby newly vacated college dormitories. And then, a new order, stat!

"Our next goal was to get as many people out as possible," noted Mak. "How many people could telecommute? How would we get equipment into these people's hands? What are some tools we can use for them to be at home yet still be online and working?" Mak added.[10]

"Over a course of not even three weeks, tens of thousands of employees in the medical system were working from home," reported Mak.[11]

From his vantage in the IT department of a regional medical facility, Mak was scrambling to keep up with the sudden and sharp transition to telemedicine. His office morphed into a studio flat with an old couch and a dorm fridge. He crashed at work so work would not crash down in a pandemic.

By April 2020, Mak reported that the use of telemedicine increased approximately ten-fold at the facility where he worked.[12] He could not find enough tablets and devices to fill the demand.

In addition, he was delivering hastily assembled instruction to medical providers who were thrust to the telemedicine platform. Tech support, which had difficulty getting on the same script, was strained by multiplying the devices in the system and by training providers and users—some of whom were hesitant or reluctant to embrace the full-on arrival of telemedicine.[13]

At a tight point in supply, he weighed converting security cameras to web-cams. Mak's message to his member check network was to expect a national shortage of tablets, webcams, and routers, as well as very limited access to tech support. Informed members updated and strengthened their technology devices before the shortage (Mak predicted) affected their areas.[14] And, hope-fully you were not in a blue area.

On March 27, 2020, Mak began accessing real-time global information system (GIS) maps on his personal phone. Areas of his county that were reporting the highest numbers of COVID-19-positive persons were displayed in darker shades of blue (figure 3.2).[15] He noted that the maps, available from the web version of the local newspaper, were addictive for a few days. Trance-like, stare, refresh, stare.

"It was great for a week! I looked at it every day. I would zoom in—look at this neighborhood right here, and then the novelty wore off. The whole place was turning blue."[16]

It was unclear to Mak as to how or if he should change his behavior when observing large blue circles (dense COVID-19 positive areas) on his phone's

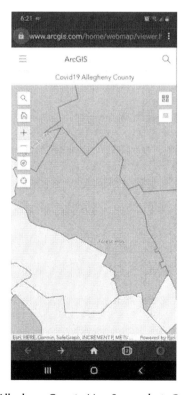

Figure 3.2 **COVID-19 Allegheny County Map Screenshot.** *Credit Charles Mak.*

navigation app. The city did not close the streets to those neighborhoods. There was not a sign that flashed, *High COVID-19 Zone —Roll Up Your Windows*. To navigate the city without going through a hue of blue would be the adult incarnation of playing The Floor is Lava.

After a week of curiosity thrills, Mak found no practical use for the superfluous information that had hacked his attention.

And, other members of his network were not reporting neighborhood "hot zones" maps.[17] Mak's observation fell into a larger basin of unique local responses to the pandemic. Other members of the same member check network, however, did find commonalities through observed local indicators.

BRYAN IN THE BRONX

A cryptozoologist and expert on the Jersey Devil who appeared on the show *Into the Unknown*, Bryan Bowden is also a life-long New Yorker who spent part of his career in Wall Street finance.[18] Bowden was bunched up in a high-rise apartment with his wife and children when COVID-19 stay-home orders rang the closing bell on the Bronx.[19] Bowden, along with Mak, contributed to the same member check group.

On the East coast, and in the country's largest city, Bowden walked his discernibly quiet neighborhood and used his phone to record what was happening around him.[20] In research circles, this type of sampling is known as *stochastic*, or random. It is simple and is a face validity check against official narratives.

As others in Bowden's member check network reported their observations, rudimentary patterns appeared of behaviors present or absent in larger populations. Individual members had a "sense" of what was happening on a larger level.

Kids are heard in the background of Bowden's recording: the city was not whispering, but it also was not *The Bronx* cacophony known to a native like Bowden. That change from baseline would have been lost to an outsider. Therefore, Bowden was informing the member check network with not only what he observed but also how those things were different from pre-pandemic baselines.[21]

On March 27, 2020, Bowden uploaded his four-minute "current face validity" video to YouTube.[22] He mentions a visit to a store earlier in the day where clerks limited capacity to twenty shoppers at a time. "There were no masks, no Lysol spray disinfectant, no bleach, no gloves" he says.[23] Bowden adds, "It's very sparse, there are some products, but things aren't getting replenished as they should be."[24]

Bowden's face validity in vivo experience was mismatched to what he expected he would find (expectation bias), "It's kind of odd. In a pandemic situation like this, you want to protect yourself, and it doesn't seem like people are protecting themselves properly."[25]

Bowden then describes human behavior he calls "The Talking Heads Dance" because "when you go into these stores, there are fewer and fewer people, everybody moves away from you like David Byrne in [the rock band] Talking Heads."[26]

Weeks later, Bowden apprised members of a perceived watershed observation. Landscape workers mulled around with their roaring blowers—chasing leaves from a nearby property.[27] Such unimportant, non-essential activity might have summoned law enforcement just weeks earlier! This was an indicator! And, other indicators were just around the corner.

In June 2020, all members reported coin shortages at stores and financial institutions occurring simultaneously with retailers requiring noncash payments. Signs appeared in windows of small, cash-dependent businesses such as gas stations: Credit Card Only. Other stores attempted to buy quarters from customers! (figure 3.3)

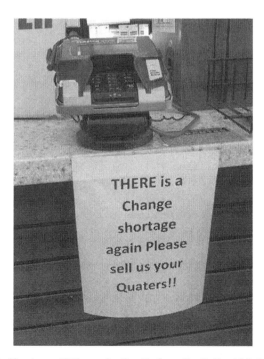

Figure 3.3   Coin Shortage at Wisconsin Gas Station. *Credit David P. Perrodin.*

Network members interpreted these indicators as omens to strengthen and expand their individual credit lines. They increased observations for bartering on marketplace websites as, per a member of the U.S. Coin Task Force, "cash is the only payment form for millions of Americans."[28]

These observed indicators allowed individuals in the member check network to prepare and adapt to changing situations during the pandemic. But how confident could they really be in their collective findings?

THE LAW OF SMALL NUMBERS—HAVING CONFIDENCE IN FINDINGS

For several decades, psychologists Daniel Kahneman and Amos Tversky studied biases that affect our decision-making processes. In 2002, their research was honored with a Nobel Prize in Economics. One of their key contributions was a paper titled, "Belief in the Law of Small Numbers."[29]

In this paper, Kahneman and Tversky define the Law of Small Numbers as the mistaken belief by researchers and laypeople alike that a small sample accurately resembles the population from which they are drawn.[30]

Let us use the example of trying to determine if a particular hotel would be a good place to stay using online reviews. The first review is a scathing condemnation about their unpleasant stay at the hotel: *Painfully sluggish check-in, rude staff, scruffy washcloth, and stale bagels passed off as a miserable continental breakfast. Never again!*

But the next review is commendatory, as are the next eight reviews. Had we read only the first review, we would have chosen other accommodations. (This tendency is known as the jump-to-conclusions bias.)

After reading the twentieth review, we trust the average rating. The first person's review was an outlier. It is not false, necessarily, but it is not representative of the larger data set of reviews which were predominantly complimentary of the facility and staff.

What else was happening during the purported "stay from hell?" Was there an unusual event in town causing staff and resources to be stretched thin for a few days? Had the person been sent to attend a contentious business meeting and attended only begrudgingly? Inclement weather? Was this traveler accustomed to luxury lodging? Was it the first day on the job for the desk clerk? What biases were in play for that reviewer?

In small data sets, misuse of outliers can lead you to incorrect conclusions and you might discover patterns where none exist (rationality bias). A member check network is a force multiplier; although not purporting to be a robust research cohort, it is nevertheless a buffer against biases and the law of small numbers. It is more than simply one or two people in the same area attempting to make sense of a sentinel chaos event.

BUILDING THE MEMBER CHECK NETWORK

"Which is more important in crisis communications—speed or accuracy? Speed is desirable and accuracy essential. If you communicate facts that are wrong, it is more damaging to your credibility than being slow."[31]

At the beginning of the COVID-19 crisis, when governors ordered people to stay home, there was no shortage of speculative reporting of National Guard deployment to patrol communities, martial law curfews, and state border checkpoints. Everything seemed to be on the table as speed was zooming past accuracy. People had an insatiable appetite for *any* news, accurate or otherwise.

Joe Dolio, the retail security executive who belonged to several industry information-sharing groups, consulted with his trade member network. Dolio's conclusion? No one knew what was happening. He persevered and made contact with a community of amateur radio enthusiasts he had become familiar with while writing his preparedness blog.

The Michigan Patriot Unified Radio Network's purpose was to share observations outside of traditional media networks—to try and be a "checks and balances" alliance to measure the on-the-ground conditions against what was being reported by the news. When COVID-19 "Stay At Home" orders were issued, the group implemented an information-sharing call every night.

During those check-ins, members described accounts of disruptions to emergency services as well as the status of infrastructure (power/utilities). They also gave firsthand assessment of visits to stores. Were customers required to use a specific entrance? Has the store's hours of operation changed? What products were selling out?

Members shared specific analysis based upon their own unique perspectives. A mechanic might note a sudden decline of cars on dealer lots in his area. What might be causing that condition? Is it the result of strong demand, low supply, or anticipation of civil unrest and potential damage to property?

As Dolio reflexively reached out to fellow retail security executives, all of them shared information from the "retail security" mindset. They observed things in similar ways, training their attention toward surveillance, management of traffic, explaining new entrance and shopping procedures to the arriving public, and access to emergency exits. They had similar training and consistent experiences, but their similar outlooks also promoted a narrow perspective vulnerable to confirmation bias.[32]

Store clerks found it difficult to communicate verbally in a masked, socially distanced environment with high background noise that included unnecessary music chirping away through the overhead speakers. Customers were confused by arrows on the floors. Was it still acceptable to tap on a watermelon to determine ripeness before selecting one? Dolio took note: seek input from people who interface in varying ways with the retail experience.

To understand population-level behavior, the preferred strategy for assembling a worthwhile information network is to look around for people from different locations and, as possible, unassociated disciplines.[33]

The U.S. military calls this "All Source Analysis," and it is an effective process to gather and receive information, as well as process it into usable intelligence. After assembling a diverse group, instruct them to use the Admiralty Scale. Practice using the Admiralty Scale with simpler tasks, such as reporting local weather, to increase inter-rater reliability.

Uncorroborated claims might cause people to panic or lose trust in information sources. They do not know what to believe, or whom to believe. If you hurl un-checked information at people, they will lose trust in you at some point. After that, you are just another talking head.

When people reported roadblocks or COVID-19 checkpoints, Dolio maintained a healthy level of skepticism, while extending trust where it was earned by empirical evidence. He paused and did not relay the information immediately. Instead, Dolio engaged in due diligence with contributors to suss out primary sources.

Nearly all of the most sensational reports were third- or fourth-hand accounts. In accordance with the Admiralty Scale, source information for these accounts was then deemed *unreliable* and information credibility was *doubtful*. Further investigation revealed the stories were hyperbole.[34]

On one occasion, Dolio was made aware of a specific National Guard COVID-19 testing checkpoint on Michigan Avenue in Dearborn Heights. The report originated from his information-sharing network.

He asked the source to describe what he had observed, the specific details of the location, vehicles, signage, people, and sequence of events. Unable to enumerate about the checkpoint, the person admitted that he had heard of the checkpoint from another source.

A second person on the sharing network reported that he had also "heard the same thing" and soon other people stated that the news of the checkpoint was confirmed by two sources. Dolio pointed out that it was heard twice, which is not the same as having been confirmed by two sources.[35]

It was still early afternoon. Dolio was nearby, and he was able to drive to the location to see firsthand what was going on.[36] In the City of Dearborn Heights, Michigan Avenue transits the city for only a few blocks, well less than a mile. Traveling the street (into Dearborn to the East and Inkster to the West) revealed that there was no National Guard or police activity.[37] It would have been simple to advance the rumor and amplify the hysteria. A twenty-minute field excursion prioritized accuracy over speed.

Dolio got it right.

After refuting a false rumor, it is vital to disseminate the results to the group in order to halt rekindling of the debunked report and to emphasize the value of protocol and use of the Admiralty Scale. This result was an opportunity to educate the group, not to shame anyone. Nobody is perfect in real time; it is difficult to recognize biases in the moment, and mistakes happen in a charged climate where pareidolia tricks our brains into seeing patterns in randomness.

Instead of debriefing in a "gotcha" style, Dolio prefers leading off with a nonjudgmental statement. "When I checked, there was no indication of a roadblock or checkpoint." With this approach, he was simply sharing his firsthand observation.

And, had the checkpoint existed before Dolio arrived at the location, the message conveyed from Dolio to the contributor was that tangible data, such as a time-stamped photo or video, brings credibility to claims. Build from this experience to improve the data collection process. All information has value, and continued sharing should be encouraged, rather than discouraged.

A similar dilemma happens when someone tells you that they have "heard something from several sources." Stop. Investigate for the original sources. The most common thing you will find, according to Dolio, is that the person who heard it from several sources actually heard it from several people who watched the one video that is now ubiquitous on the Internet.

In other words, there is only one root source, not several. If the source of the information is unclear, the following benign request might provide insight about the person's process for obtaining data: "Help me to understand how you learned about this incident."

Dolio received a video clip from someone claiming to be an "inside source."[38] This "inside source" specified, "My neighbor got this in an email from his son." That is not an inside source. That is at least fourth-hand information. This guy (4th) is reading an email he got from his neighbor (3rd), from the neighbor's son (2nd), reporting some other information (hopefully a firsthand account). The original source is notably distal from the person breaking the news. Dolio was not able to trace back to the original source. According to the Admiralty Scale, the source reliability was *reliability cannot be judged* and the information credibility was *truth cannot be judged.*

Another lesson from this example is to obtain metadata, which is data that provides information about other data. For a photo, metadata might contain the type of camera used, camera setting, size of image, location of image, and the date and time the image was taken. It would also attribute ownership to the photo. Was it captured by a person or excerpted from surveillance footage?

When multiple videos, photos, documents, and field notes are submitted to the primary collector, metadata identifies provenance, or the chronology of the location or custody of important objects or events. Metadata is particularly useful when curating stories and images submitted by member checks. It answers the questions: what, when, where, why, who, which, and how.

Dolio recommends capturing images with the Solocator camera app for phones. "You can easily email photos from the app with compass bearing, house elevation, the time taken, GPS coordinates and links to iOS maps or Google maps."[39]

When local media was reporting that Detroit hospital emergency rooms (ERs) were overwhelmed, and that information was shared as factual on the network, Dolio grabbed a cell phone equipped with the Solocator app and spent a day unobtrusively visiting local ERs throughout Metro Detroit. He snapped photos of empty ER parking areas and no waiting lines at entrances.[40]

Dolio's contributions, in tandem with similar firsthand reports from others, were able to be authenticated with location and time, and quelled the overrun-ER rumors within the group (figure 3.4). Note, Dolio was not reporting what was happening inside the hospitals. He was observing parking areas, entrances, and lobbies—the same areas appearing in local news clips.

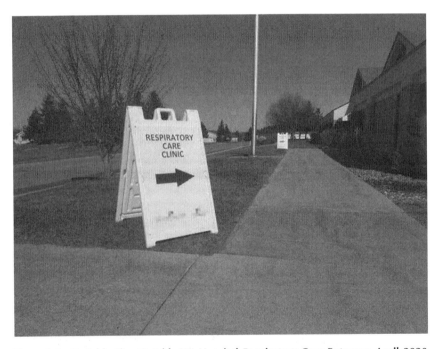

Figure 3.4   Portable Sign Outside WI Hospital Respiratory Care Entrance, April 2020. *Credit David P. Perrodin for photo and credit Drew Baye for pixelating the name of the hospital on the signs.*

In spite of efforts from contributors to obtain and document firsthand information, there continued to be multiple announcements of checkpoints and roadblocks. Other members rushed to verify the information, only to find free-flowing traffic each time. The errant claims were overwhelmingly provided from one contributor. Frustrated by "false alarms," a faction in the group's leadership sought to remove the unreliable member from the network.

Dolio advocated to keep him, and to extend coaching to increase his fidelity of situational observation, to suppress reporting of mere opinions, and to apply the Admiralty Scale. The contributor was overwhelmed, but learning. He had not practiced gathering and communicating field information. It was his first pandemic, after all.

Demonstrating empathy to this person conveyed to all members that the group will pull together during the crisis. That message prevents people from measuring or withdrawing their participation due to apprehension of consequences for being inaccurate.

It was Dolio's sticking recommendation that the group would continue to verify this contributor's claims, while listing, at least in the interim, the information as unconfirmed and unreliable.[41]

This situation was a contemporary version of *The Boy Who Cried Wolf* from *Aesop's Fables*.[42] Yes, the boy falsely cried wolf many times, but one time, the wolf was actually there, and wreaked havoc on the sheep because no one believed the boy anymore.

Tragedy could have been avoided if the village had continued to verify the boy's story. Accept the information and attempt to verify it from another source. That second step, attempting to verify information, has long been a shortcoming for previous generations.

On October 28, 1938, many Americans believed they were being invaded by Martians. This erroneous belief was the result of a Halloween stunt orchestrated by Orson Welles in which he adapted H. G. Wells's *War of the Worlds* to the radio and then broadcast the play as though it was actually happening.[43]

"A few short weeks before this broadcast, millions of listeners had kept their radios tuned for the latest news from a Europe apparently about to go to war."[44] Radio listeners therefore had a preexisting expectation bias toward catastrophically bad news.

In the weeks that followed, Psychology professor Howard Cantril of Princeton University and colleagues interviewed people to try and understand their reactions to the broadcast.[45] Of those that mistook the radio play as a live news report, almost none of them tuned to another station where they would have quickly found that life was completely normal.

Even more concerning, "People who were frightened or disturbed by the news often hastened to telephone friends or relatives."[46] Rather than attempting to verify the news of the invasion, these individuals were more concerned with spreading the terror-inducing information as quickly as possible. In chapter 2, we learned from Nikolai, the Russian cyclist, that it is critically important to gather additional information before sharing a story headline without the rest of the story.

The key to reducing panic is to report back to your network that which has been determined to have been false or misleading information. If you do not, everyone else in the network who heard the original false or misleading information is then re-sharing the false information as fact.

A note about unconfirmed information: It is exactly that. It is not confirmed. It may still be true and it may still be false. Keep the information, but be very careful about sharing it, especially in today's digital information society. If you decide to share it, be very clear about its status as unconfirmed.

For this same reason, whenever someone reports information to you and then provides a conclusion, ask them why they came to that conclusion. An example of this principle came from a contributor who conveyed to Dolio's group that a primary grocery store was limiting the number of customers.

But in fact, the 75-foot line outside the store was caused by implementation of social distancing requirements. Customers were adjusting to standing on the "X" taped on the pavement, and then hopping forward to the next "X." It was like hopscotch for adults. The flow of customers into the store was clunky due to the change in entrance protocol. And, the store was not limiting the number of shoppers.

When the process is performed correctly, people separate their opinion (the conclusion) from the information. This step is vital, and one that we often overlook in modern communications. In this example, it was the difference between people learning a new behavior and a change in policy that might limit people's access to food and essential supplies.

Confirmation bias also plays a role in awareness versus panic. When someone believes something to be true, they will seek sources that agree with them and immediately refute or discount sources that do not agree as "biased." To combat this phenomenon, seek the truth of the issue, rather than confirmation of your opinion or position.

In any investigation, the goal is to find the truth, not to confirm suspicions or predetermined positions. If you approach panic-inducing situations with that attitude, you will arrive at awareness, rather than panic. Your initial assumptions and conclusions may not always be correct.

For example, imagine watching a professional baseball game on TV and texting your attending-in-person friend, "Stadium is packed! Hope the concession lines aren't a mile long!" Seconds later, they respond with a wide-angle selfie from a bleacher seat, "What are you talking about? This place is practically empty!"

On July 23, 2020, Fox Sports posted a thirty-seven-second video to its Twitter account demonstrating how it would place thousands of virtual life-like fans in the stands of major league stadiums.[47] "Fox Sports producers will be able to control things like how full the virtual 'crowds' are for a given game, what weather fans are dressed for, and what percentage of the crowd will be home fans versus away."[48] The crowds appeared strikingly authentic and would be indiscernible from real crowds to most TV viewers.

That snippet was both incredible and chilling at the same time. What other real-world scenarios could be "hacked" to distort crowd density? Political rallies, protests, lines outside stores? Is there an app for that?

Member checks will become even more important in the future as a countermeasure to Internet bots spamming out algorithm falsehoods, deep fakes, and virtual avatars that are able to create the illusion of crowds. Human networks will be an indispensable defense to resist well-crafted disinformation.

Three Keys to Building an Efficient Member Check Network

- **Include people from various occupations and locations.** An efficient network includes diversity of perspective and interests.
- **Provide metadata to ensure accurate descriptions.** All information that you receive via your network should be time-stamped and saved, along with its eventual status of either confirmed, proven false, or unconfirmed. You can do this either digitally or in written form. As you read in chapter 1, be cognizant of offloading crucial data to cloud-based storage because as exemplified during the unrest in places from Belarus to Myanmar in 2020, governments or rogue actors can suspend Internet access.
- **Maintain data in multiple locations so it can be accessed during Internet service disruptions.** A piece of information you gather today may only become relevant much later. Also, if you have the data, including the meta information and its status, saved somewhere locally (such as within an Access database), you can run a quick search of your own database and quickly either confirm or refute data.

NOTES

1. Zheng, Min, Jessecae K. Marsh, Jeffrey V. Nickerson and Samantha Kleinberg. "How Causal Information Affects Decisions." *Cognitive Research* 5, no. 6 (2020). doi: 10.1186/s41235-020-0206-z.

2. Besombes, Jerome, Vincent Nimier, and Laurence Cholvy. "Information Evaluation in Fusion Using Information Correlation." Paper presented at the 12th International Conference on Information Fusion. Seattle, 2009. Joseph, John, and Jeff

Corkill. "Information Evaluation: How One Group of Intelligence Analysts Go about The Task." Edith Cowan University. Australian Security and Intelligence Conference. January 1, 2011, 100. https://ro.ecu.edu.au/cgi/viewcontent.cgi?article=1019&context=asi.

3. Jardine, Cynthia G., Franziska U. Boerner, Amanda D. Boyd, and S. Michelle Driedger. "The More the Better? A Comparison of the Information Sources Used by the Public During Two Infectious Disease Outbreaks." *PLoS ONE* 10, no. 10 (2015): 1. Doi: 10.1371/journal.pone.0140028.

4. Jardine et al., *The More the Better?*, 4.

5. Ibid., 15.

6. Ibid., 1.

7. Charles Mak, "Face Validity From Pittsburgh." Interview by David P. Perrodin. *The Safety Doc Podcast*, May 5, 2020. https://tinyurl.com/SDP133-AUDIO.

8. Mak, *Face Validity From Pittsburgh.*

9. Ibid.

10. Ibid.

11. Ibid.

12. Ibid.

13. Ibid.

14. Ibid.

15. Ibid.

16. Ibid.

17. Ibid.

18. Bryan Bowden, "Jersey Devil." Into the Unknown (TV Series). March 16, 2020. https://www.imdb.com/title/tt11991002/?ref_=nm_flmg_tk_1.

19. Bryan Bowden, "NYC Pandemic Epicenter Face Validity: Protecting Your Right to Privacy." Interview by David P. Perrodin. *The Safety Doc Podcast.* April 9, 2020. https://tinyurl.com/SDP128-AUDIO.

20. Bowden, *NYC Pandemic Epicenter Face Validity.*

21. Ibid.

22. Bryan Bowden, "Bowden V-Log 3/26/29 Current Status Face Validity." YouTube. March 27, 2020. https://youtu.be/Ry7fi3pGCZY.

23. Bowden, *NYC Pandemic Epicenter Face Validity.*

24. Ibid.

25. Ibid.

26. Ibid.

27. Ibid.

28. Walker, Hannah vL. "Statement from the U.S. Coin Task Force on the Coin Circulation Issue." U.S. Coin Task Force. May 18, 2020. https://getcoinmoving.org/.

29. Tversky, Amos and Daniel Kahneman. "Belief in the Law of Small Numbers." *Psychological Bulletin* 76, no. 2 (1971): 105–110. doi: 10.1037/h0031322.

30. Tversky and Kahneman, *Belief in the Law of Small Numbers,* 105–110.

31. Caesar-Gordon, Andrew. "Speed Versus Accuracy in Crisis Comms." PR Week. October 28, 2015. https://www.prweek.com/article/1357205/speed-versus-accuracy-cirsis-comms.

32. Joe Dolio, "Assessing the Situation, Body Cams, Mustering the Member Checks." Interview by David P. Perrodin. *The Safety Doc Podcast.* July 8, 2020. https://tinyurl.com/SDP142-AUDIO.

33. Dolio, *Assessing the Situation.*

34. Ibid.

35. Ibid.

36. Ibid.

37. Ibid.

38. Ibid.

39. Solocator. "About Solocator." Civi Corp Pty Limited. 2021. https://solocator.com.

40. Dolio, *Assessing the Situation.*

41. Ibid.

42. Ibid.

43. Welles, Orson. "War of the Worlds." The Mercury Theatre on Air. Aired October 30, 1938. https://archive.org/details/OrsonWellesMrBruns.

44. Cantril, Hadley, Hazel Gaudet, and Herta Herzog. *The Invasion From Mars: A Study in the Psychology of Panic with the Complete Script of the Famous Orson Welles Broadcast* (Princeton: Princeton University Press, 1940), 68.
    https://canvas.harvard.edu/files/2618975/download?download_frd=1&verifier =0lplYVHsuaePIRWmerzmzugBkAyjMWU1TvQKDPj3.

45. Cantril, Gaudet, and Herzog, *The Invasion From Mars*, 70.

46. Ibid., 83.

47. Fox Sports. [@FoxSports.] "No Fans? Not on FOX Sports. Thousands of Virtual Fans Will Attend FOX's MLB Games This Saturday." Twitter. July 23, 2020. https://twitter.com/FOXSports/status/1286281346390740993.

48. Gartenberg, Chaim. "How Fox Sports Will Use Virtual Fans Created in Unreal Engine to Fill Empty Stadiums in MLB Broadcasts. Real Sports, Fake Fans." The Verge. July 25, 2020. https://www.theverge.com/2020/7/25/21336017/fox-sports -baseball-virtual-fans-epic-unreal-engine-empty-stadiums-mlb.

Chapter 4

Finite Voltage

THE BREAKING POINT

Everyone has a breaking point. For the purpose of this book, that breaking point will be referred to as *finite voltage*. It is a term borrowed from electrical circuitry which describes the pressure that pushes electrons (current) through a conducting loop.

We can plug a lamp and a laptop into an outlet without any problem. Add a vacuum cleaner, microwave, and guitar amplifier to that same outlet and the current flow will eventually overload the circuit—perhaps as you unleash the powerful bass riff.

In a home, overloading the electrical circuit heats up the wires and trips a circuit breaker or blows a fuse, shutting off the circuit. The remedy is often simple and quick. Unplug things and then snap the breaker back to the "on" position or replace the melted fuse with a fresh one. Good to go.

Humans approach finite voltage during periods of intense mental stress. This overload can be caused by a sudden, single event such as the unexpected death of a loved one. It can also be caused by a gradual compounding of stress contributors—the progressive plugging of more things into the outlet. For example, you might reach finite voltage after you lose your job, then divorce after spousal abandonment, followed by the engine blowing out on your old truck. Crossing the threshold of finite voltage manifests as mental collapse and being unable to function in everyday life. Suicide is the ultimate manifestation of an individual reaching finite voltage.

Finite voltage occurs on both the individual and population level. Humans' differing resilience to pressure means that some will arrive at finite voltage sooner or later than others, but most civilians will encounter finite voltage approximately ninety days into an extended chaos situation.

Lack of moderate stress for long periods of time would mean that if change were to occur, regular levels of stress would be perceived as more difficult than they actually are. People adjust and handle the pressure, or the pressure overwhelms them in something known as a *wet bulb effect.*

WET BULBS

Your phone buzzes. It is a push alert from the newspaper you trust, about the governor's upcoming press conference on COVID-19 (figure 4.1). Another alert comes in an hour later: case and death numbers and summary guidance from the press conference.

The phone buzzes a third time. It is an emergency alert ordered by the governor; if you had somehow missed his comments earlier.

On your way home, a dynamic messaging sign on the freeway encourages you to "mask up." Your televised football game is interrupted by misty-eyed celebrities urging that "we're all in this together." The 11 o'clock news will offer the very latest.

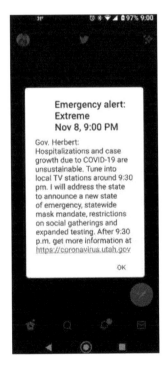

Figure 4.1   Utah Emergency Alert Phone Push Notification, November 8, 2020. *Credit Robert Peterson.*

No amount of muted words or thoughtful curation will keep updates out of your social media feed. There is no escape. And we would not have it any other way. We bask in the warm glow.

A wet bulb temperature is taken when you wrap an ambient-temperature thermometer bulb in a wet muslin fabric, exposing it to air flow to promote evaporation, and then measure the difference in temperature. When the air is hot and humid, evaporation is stifled and the wet bulb and dry bulb measurements will be close—too close for comfort. We are saturated, swimming in sweat, and overheating.

Cyclists, like Nikolai Razouvaev, rely on the wet bulb measurement to inform their decision to take the bicycle out on a hot and humid day.[1] What can be done to cool down? Perhaps lighter clothing, extra water, frequent breaks, easier terrain, or postponing the outing for a time with a lower wet bulb reading. But what if you do not have an option? What if you must race?

In a global pandemic, at the height of the Information Age, we are all wet bulbs, spinning away. We are not just wet, we are soaked. And we chose this situation for ourselves.

The U.S. Department of Defense defines *Time on Target* as "the actual time at which munitions impact the target."[2] Military commanders set their watches to it. If the plan works, when the time comes and the attacks arrive, the enemy is bombarded. Eighty years ago, during World War II, *Time on Target* was an achievement of strategy. It was the work of trained military minds.

These days we train the targets on ourselves. We opt in to news push alerts. And we could opt out of emergency alerts, if we so chose. But in both cases, we have decided that the risk of saturation is tolerable compared to the alternative, fear of missing out. The velocity of information is too great to remove ourselves from the equation.

In April 2020, a couple accused of shooting a man at his suburban Detroit home were tracked by police to another suburb a short drive away. Police found them by pinging their cell phones.[3]

On our torus, our cell phones are too close to the center of our routines to navigate life without them. Our phones are a daily test of our finite voltage. And yet we cannot, and will not, go without them. Even when they burn us out. Even when they lead the police right to us.

Identifying our approaching breaking point is the first step. The next step is changing behavior to avoid finite voltage.

BREAKING PARKINSON'S LAW IN CHICAGO

Prior to 2020, Aaron Sawyer's Redline VR, a virtual reality club and bar in the Ravenswood neighborhood of Chicago, was doing great business.

His mega-computers, 3D game configurations, and 360-degree immersive goggles and haptic wearables were something that people could not get at home. He offered the best zombie-battling experience in the city. So much so that Sawyer considered opening a second location.[4]

Then the pandemic hit.

Chicago city government started deciding which businesses were "essential," and thus allowed to operate, and which were not. Redline VR was not deemed "essential."

Under Mayor Lori Lightfoot's plan, Redline VR was allowed to reopen in phase four[5] at 25 percent capacity. There was no phase five. There was no revenue coming into the business. So Sawyer pivoted. Again and again.[6]

Parkinson's Law states that "work expands so as to fill the time available for its completion."[7] Linda Stone, the consultant who has studied attention behavior, found that during the pandemic, people were checking work emails "at all hours of the night," as their homes became their workplace.[8]

At the outset of the pandemic, many people left their office on a Friday, began working remotely the following Monday, and did not return to their offices. Many still have no return date in sight, and a significant number of positions have become permanently remote.

Getting out of the home, and into an office setting, became an attractive option for some people. At home, the roles of spouse and mother and caregiver all intersect with the workday.

Work now fills the physical space once reserved for family and relaxation. The mind is not always able to differentiate between the two.

It took several pivots before Sawyer realized that Redline VR could be of value for such workers. In mid-April 2020, Sawyer resorted to a GoFundMe campaign to keep his business afloat financially.[9] But goodwill donations are not sustainable as a business plan. Redline VR was but one of many businesses in Chicago affected by the government's restrictions.

By month's end Redline VR was serving take-out cocktails. If people could not come in to play virtual reality games, they could come in to buy drinks to go, with virtual reality gear available to use as they waited.

"Cocktails-to-go sometimes turned into $200 in arcade sales," Sawyer said.[10] But that did not happen with the frequency needed to sustain a business.

In May and June, Sawyer changed course again. Redline VR needed regular revenue. Sawyer decided to market Redline VR as office space. "I said, 'I gotta be a phase three business,'" Sawyer said. "Offices are a phase three business. The license to have an office is just $250."[11]

Redline VR rebranded to offer rented office space, at just fifteen dollars for the day. Curtains and separators were put up so people could keep their social distance and have a work space of their own, away from home and family (figure 4.2).

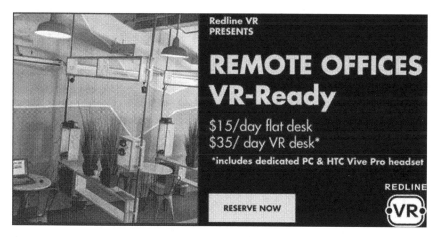

Figure 4.2   Redline VR Remote Office Advertisement. *Credit Aaron Sawyer.*

In Redline's pivot to office space, the rollout was not smooth. The very first day, fumes from a neighboring business forced Sawyer to close shop early and refund the one and only paying customer.[12]

But, over time, rentals picked up a bit, as people looking to restore the feel and routine of the work day would use the Redline VR office space to draw a clear line between work and home.

In July, 2020, about 1 in 4 employed people teleworked or worked from home for pay because of the coronavirus disease pandemic. These data refer to employed people who teleworked or worked at home for pay at some point in the last 4 weeks specifically because of the coronavirus disease pandemic. This measure does not include those whose telework was unrelated to the pandemic, such as employed people who worked entirely from home before the pandemic.[13]

"I'm just helping people get out of their house, away from their kids and spouse," Sawyer said in an interview.[14] People came to Redline VR to restore some of the pre-pandemic separation and balance between home and work.

And with the day paid for and the arcade gear nearby, one thing sometimes led to another. "In phase three, people would ask if [they] could [play on the machines], and I would say yes," Sawyer said. "Because anything can happen in an office."[15]

When phase four eventually came, and Redline VR was allowed to operate as an arcade, at 25 percent capacity, business actually *declined*. "Phase four has not been successful to me," Sawyer said.[16] With restaurants and bars again open to the dining and drinking public, Redline VR lost ground to them.

There was one more pivot left. Sawyer called it his "Hail Mary." Redline VR would market the physical nature of the virtual reality games as a fitness experience. Some of the games are so physical Sawyer warns people out on dates that they are likely to get sweaty playing them. "At 7 p.m., that's a bug, but at 7 a.m., that's a feature," Sawyer explained.[17]

Rather than merely seek customers, Redline VR would sign up members, allowing it to better handle unplanned disruptions in the future. "We're taking a hint from the gym in that way," said Sawyer.[18]

A friend who owns a gym nearby once complained he was down 30 percent revenue during the pandemic, but "I was down one hundred percent," Sawyer revealed.[19]

A three-month membership commitment to Redline VR costs the same as five hours on the arcade machines would, if paid for individually. By letting Redline VR be whatever its customers needed from it that day—an arcade, a bar, a meeting room, an office, a gym—Sawyer has been able to stay in business, rather than shutter his doors.

During a pandemic that has turned home into office and office into home, and blurred the lines between the two, Redline VR offered a taste of the old normal, when people left home to work and returned home after work.

With his business on the wrong end of "essential," Sawyer changed again and again to survive, in ways that honored both the government's orders and the marketplace. Sawyer did not have a plan for an once-in-a-lifetime global pandemic. But because he was willing to think his way through it, again and again, he was able to survive and eventually hit on a business model that worked.

Before COVID-19, Redline VR had customers. Now it has members.

DR. JOHN APPEL, WORLD WAR II, AND
THE LESSON OF FINITE VOLTAGE

"If you gotta go, you gotta go."

To look at pictures of the Normandy invasion on D-Day, one attributes to the American troops landing on the beach, swimming and running headlong into gunfire, an admirable certainty of mission. Surely, the men rushing into gunfire knew that success would mean their children, and perhaps their grandchildren, could live free. Surely, with murderous foes such as Adolf Hitler (and the Imperial Japanese military in the Pacific theater), failure was unthinkable.

But when American psychiatrist Dr. John Appel looked into the eyes of would-be war fighters at draft intake and asked them why they wanted to pursue military service, their answers concerned him. The draftees did not, in fact, "want" military service. They had been drafted into it. And they had no problem saying so.

"If you gotta go, you gotta go," the draftees would say, Dr. Appel recalled decades later in a 1999 journal article called "Fighting Fear: The Role of Psychiatrists in World War II."[20] "Their resigned, apathetic reply to my question hardly seemed conducive to effective performance, let alone to their mental health," Dr. Appel wrote.[21]

After the December 7, 1941, Japanese attack on the Pearl Harbor military base in Hawaii, America became a participant in World War II, after years of sitting on the sideline. "Did these young men leap to our defense?" Dr. Appel questioned. "No. They were not volunteering; they had been drafted."[22]

Dr. Appel decided that his part in the war effort would be to help soldiers prevent the mental breakdowns that are disqualifying from further military service. "It came to me that perhaps I could help prevent soldiers from breaking down, rather than try to treat them after they had done so," Dr. Appel recalled.[23] "My assignment was to prevent the seven million men in the Army from having nervous breakdowns."[24] Dr. Appel enlisted as a lieutenant in the U.S. Army and served as Chief of the preventive psychiatry branch of the U.S. Surgeon General's Office during the war.

Prior to World War II, the common belief in the U.S. military was that some people burn out during war, and some people do not. The ones who do, the "weaklings" and "neurotics," had to be weeded out from the ranks.

"The military wisdom of the day held that normal soldiers did not break down, that only neurotics did," Dr. Appel noted.[25] "This belief had led to the policy of screening 'weaklings' out of the Army."[26]

The results of those screenings were costly to the war effort. About 12 percent of the rejections at induction stations were attributed to "psychiatric" reasons. And "psychiatric cases accounted for more than a third of all casualties being shipped home from overseas," Dr. Appel observed.[27]

Dr. Appel took a softer stance: What if some people who would normally be screened out just needed a break? What if they had simply reached their finite voltage in the moment, but had more value to offer down the line? What if there is a level before final, forever burnout, and men could be temporarily pulled from duty before reaching it?

Dr. Appel concluded: "This was an issue of tremendous significance. If normal men could break, it meant that the problem of military psychiatry involved not just a small segment of abnormal individuals but the whole Army."[28]

Efforts to improve mental health, Dr. Appel wrote, "would have to focus not on the soldiers, but the soldiers' environment, identifying the stresses in it and attempting to reduce them."[29] Dr. Appel ordered psychiatrists to work in the field with soldiers, and they were also assigned as advisers to commanders.

After discovering what sounded like low morale and a disinterest in the war mission, Dr. Appel's first thought was to use propaganda to remind warf-ighters what was at stake. "My plan was to use mass media to show Hitler's and Japan's intent—and ability—to conquer the United States along with the rest of the world. I reasoned that if this were done effectively, it would make the troops angry and eager—in short, motivated."[30]

Why We Fight, and the Limits of Propaganda

Dr. Appel was part of a team of mental health professionals, including Dr. Theodor Seuss Geisel—better known as children's author, Dr. Seuss—who worked with Hollywood filmmakers to produce seven propaganda films called "Why We Fight."[31]

These films would be shown to enlisted men and were designed to pull their heartstrings such that they would willingly embrace the hell that is war. "The purpose of these films," explained a disclaimer at the beginning of each video, "is to give factual information as to the causes, the events leading up to our entry into the war, and the principles for which we are fighting."[32]

This approach misread the problem.

War was a "democratic surround" all its own, as all-encompassing as it got. Tours of duty longer than six months were common. The men who invaded Normandy did not lack for motivation. It was not the individual mindset of the soldier that needed fixing, Dr. Appel learned, but rather the endless physi-cal and mental demands placed on enlisted men.

A soldier new to the front line faced several potential outcomes, most of them bad: death, injury, or endless war, the better part of a year spent fight-ing. Few breaks, if any. "The only way out was death, injury, or war's end," Dr. Appel wrote.[33]

This untenable situation created the morale problem, not any lack of knowledge about the dangers of fascism. Morale is tough to come by when the conditions and demands of life are demoralizing and will not change.

Dr. Appel's team noted the prevalence of "old sergeant's syndrome" among people a year or two into their service. When they would turn up in field hospitals, Dr. Appel wrote, these soldiers would tell doctors that they were the "old man" in the unit, or that the few old men left would soon join him in treatment.[34] "The old sergeant syndrome was a fairly consis-tent constellation of attitudes and symptoms occurring in well-motivated, previously efficient soldiers as a result of the chronic and progressive breakdown of the normal defenses against anxiety over long periods of combat."[35]

Propaganda films beating the drums of war were less effective than new policies that gave fighters breaks from the front line, gave infantrymen a tangible, physical reward for their risky service, and the creation of combat pay.

The infantryman, the front line fighter, lowest in the hierarchy, arguably had it the worst, carrying the heavy duty of direct war fighting while taking orders from seemingly everybody else. The infantryman, Dr. Appel wrote, "saw himself as underappreciated, as the low man on the totem pole, the sucker."[36] If infantrymen felt embarrassed by their station, the Army would have to show, publicly, that their role in the war was respected, Dr. Appel argued to military brass.

The bosses listened.

On Dr. Appel's recommendation, infantrymen were given special blue badges to wear on their uniforms. They came in two forms, Dr. Appel explained: "Plain for infantrymen who had not yet fought and embellished with a silver wreath once the wearer had seen action."[37] These badges could only be given to infantrymen. Not officers, not Special Forces, not anyone else but the grunts. Just that quickly, the infantrymen were "suckers" no more.

They were soldiers who played an important role, and that role was recognized through special insignia by the U.S. Army. It could not be gotten any other way but earning it. By war's end, tours of duty for infantrymen were capped at 180 days, an "Army-wide policy" that would continue during the Korean and Vietnam Wars, Dr. Appel noted.[38]

The power of images such as special insignia also translated to other forms of media, as well. While Capra was attempting to motivate young men with "Why We Fight" films, the military knew a compelling reason why men fought—and that was for attractive women back home.

World War II in 1941 was the golden age of [sexy] pinups. For the first time in history, the US military unofficially sanctioned the creation and distribution of pinup pictures, magazines and calendars to troops in order to raise morale and remind young men what they were fighting for. [P]inup posters adorned servicemen's lockers, the walls of barracks, and even the sides of planes.[39]

Considered risqué by some, the pinup girls became an important source of morale building for the U.S. military. That the use of pinup art was not officially recognized did nothing to diminish its importance.

What improved morale on the front lines of World War II was not rah-rah motivational techniques or propaganda films, but basic signs of respect, acknowledgments of basic motivations for young men, and policy changes that acknowledge all are people susceptible to burnout, eventually. Even when they are fighting Hitler.

This susceptibility does not make soldiers weak, or neurotic, and it does not mean they are burned out forever. It just means they are human.

Findings on Finite Voltage: The Lessons of World War II

- **Everybody breaks down eventually.** After 200 days of war in the Mediterranean theater, 90 percent of a regiment would be killed, wounded, captured, mentally collapse, or found to be missing in action.[40]
- **Breakdowns are contagious.** Warfighters between days 200 and 240 of combat were "jittery under shell fire and so overly cautious" that they "demoralized" newer men on the front lines. Psychiatric breakdowns were highest where the most men were killed.[41]
- **Breaks prevent breakdowns.** Dr. Appel observed that the British got 400 days out of their men on the Italian front lines compared to half that for the Americans. The British would pull fighters out of duty within twelve days, for a rest period of four days, while Americans were then serving anywhere from twenty to eighty days without relief.[42]
- **Badge of respect.** Once the blue combat patches had begun to be worn by infantrymen, commanders started to notice an increase in pride among the soldiers wearing them. Dr. Appel believed that the badges raised morale and increased soldiers' resilience.
- **Finite voltage beats forever burnout.** Using these approaches, people with psychiatric disorders, and those with under 200 days of fighting, could eventually be returned to active duty. But someone who fully burned out was done forever as a warfighter and was often unable to reintegrate into civilian life successfully.

CLAY MARTIN, DEATH BY DR. PEPPER, AND THE GOD COMPLEX

The sniper took his post on the roof of a building. He aimed at his target. And realized he had no bullets in his SR-25 rifle. This was not a training exercise. This was war. And the sniper was unprepared to do his work. "It was frightening, to catch myself slipping like that," said that sniper, Clay Martin.[43]

Observational skills and preparedness are essential tools for a sniper. Forgetting to load one's secondary weapon after "firing it dry" the night before was the act of a rookie.

But Martin was not a rookie. He was a Green Beret, a veteran of the U.S. Army Special Forces, and before that a Marine. In the time since, he has penned *Concrete Jungle: A Green Beret's Guide to Urban Survival.*

"That's day-one stuff: you put bullets back in your gun," Martin said. "But the next night I got up on the roof, and there were no bullets in my SR-25."[44] As a sniper, part of Martin's training included memory and observational drills designed to make such lapses impossible.

The work of the sniper—shooting people from long distances—is precise. Facing camouflaged targets trying to remain hidden, the slightest movement can offer opportunity. Snipers are trained to notice everything. "There are hours and hours of training devoted to ruining your day if you missed a small detail," Martin said in a June 2020 guest appearance on *The Safety Doc Podcast*.[45]

"You'll be walking somewhere, like to eat lunch," Martin said. "You'll be asked later, 'what was on the sidewalk?' And you better know it."[46] Trainees would also play Kim's Game. Several items will be laid out on a table, and the trainees will have a short time frame to observe and remember them. Then the items are removed, and the trainees are tested on what they saw.

The training is made more intense over time. Trainees are given less time to review the items, or greater time duration between seeing the items and being quizzed on them—perhaps after an entire day of hard training. Or both.[47]

"It opens your brain up to start processing more," Martin said of the observational training.[48] Those who cannot excel are weeded out of the program. Kim's Game has stood between many would-be Special Forces fighters and their dreams.

Army Special Forces fighters also go through Robin Sage training in North Carolina. Military members from Fort Bragg play-act as opposition fighters. Civilians partake as role-players. Robin Sage training covers fifteen counties of ground and is highly orchestrated with local law enforcement.

Candidates are placed in an environment of political instability characterized by armed conflict, forcing soldiers to analyze and solve problems to meet the challenges of this "real-world" training.[49] Friend? Foe? Civilian? Actor? For the entirety of the two-week program, the final test before they start work in the Special Forces, trainees cannot take anything they see for granted.

Robin Sage is one of the many trainings Martin was exposed to over the years. Despite it all, despite the wartime setting, despite the soldier's trained hypervigilance, Martin had reached finite voltage, and burned out. And in that state, he was as susceptible to a rookie mistake as anyone else.

Years prior, in October 2001, during a USMC sniper training in Quantico, Virginia, when he actually was a rookie, Martin learned his lesson on hypervigilance the hard way. The training mission was to achieve a sniper shot at the platoon sergeant and retrieve the briefcase he was carrying. Inside there was a mortar tube with food and other supplies.

With Halloween approaching, the sergeant had planned a spooky surprise for the trainee snipers. The group took the mortar tube back to its "hide sight," where snipers rest, and broke it open. After eating barely edible foodstuffs for five days, the snipers had retrieved a cache of honey buns and other sugary treats. Score! The last thing inside was a Dr. Pepper bottle. "That sounds absolutely fantastic," Martin thought at the time.[50]

But the bottle would not pull from the tube easily. It had to be given a hard yank. Instead of offering Dr. Pepper's "unique blend of twenty-three flavors," the bottle was a decoy concealing a tear gas grenade—which had just been yanked open. Hard. "It falls in the middle of us and sets my ghillie suit on fire," Martin said. "That was a lesson. You have to treat everything like a booby trap."[51]

In addition to being susceptible to rookie mistakes, reaching finite voltage can also give way to something known as the God Complex.

BEWARE OF THE GOD COMPLEX

In the fictitious HBO series *The Wire*, homicide detectives in the Baltimore Police Department worked long hours. When one of the detectives fell asleep on the job, a colleague would cut off their necktie, and add it to the "cut necktie mausoleum," as one character called it.[52]

Falling asleep at work was a testament to the long hours required of homicide detectives. Working forty-eight hours straight on a new, hot case is not unusual in that world. Having a necktie meant the detective was suffering the tortures of the righteous. The guys working in the pawn shop unit did not work long enough or hard enough to be caught sleeping on the job. Only the elite.

Martin said the reconnaissance Marines had a similar acknowledgment of burnout, called a "Cracked Board." Sometime around ninety days into their tour, a soldier would have a shortcoming of action or temperament that indicated they had "cracked." Their name would then be added to the "Cracked Board," Martin said.[53]

"The instinct at first is to avoid getting on that board," Martin said.[54] For a soldier's name to appear on that board was a reminder to one and all that finite voltage does not respect anyone. Everybody cracks eventually. No matter how skilled or experienced.

Martin noticed two threats to soldiers who had been in the field a long time. One is cracking. The other is the God Complex. As Martin describes it, the God Complex is when a fighter, "after surviving so much stuff that should have killed them, thinks they cannot be killed."[55]

During the Global War on Terror, Martin said many soldiers who were veterans in the war, those who had served eight and nine tours, would make "tactically stupid" moves. Sometimes those mistakes resulted in death. "A fair number of guys have gone out that way," Martin said.[56]

Believing they were invincible led to making preventable and foreseeable mistakes. Hubris cured by death is permanent. The God Complex can be fatally dangerous.

COVID-19: Locking Down and Opening Up

Martin wryly jokes that his family had "an incredible 2020, even by 2020 standards."[57] A house fire in late January cost the family its home. A week later, Martin was in the hospital with blood clots down his entire right arm, and in both lungs. He was hospitalized for ten days, all told. Oh, and COVID-19 was fast approaching America's shores.

There was no time for a God Complex; Martin was acutely aware of the serious risks a respiratory illness would pose, given a double pulmonary embolism. "It was scary for anybody with lung issues. We had to seal off," Martin said. "Nothing in or out for thirty days."[58]

With two young children, ages two and four years old, the Martins faced constant, repeated questions about where their toys were. It was the kids' way of asking when life would get back to normal. But as Martin began member-checking his network, he found that hospitals were not overwhelmed. At one point previously, Martin had wondered if COVID-19 would kill 20 percent of the global population.

About sixty days in, after the first wave of the pandemic, he realized it would not. "Ninety days in, we were fully convinced this was no worse than the flu," Martin said.[59]

Further study found that most of the people dying were high-risk, and already in poor health. Fitness can be the difference between life and death in an acute trauma situation, Martin explained. "If you're a more fit human being, with more cardiovascular endurance, you'll survive a gunshot that would have killed an obese person," Martin continued. "Because once they have that trauma to their chest, all that extra weight puts them under. They can't survive on that little bit of oxygen, where a high-performance athlete can."[60]

With Martin recovering from his health issues, and the COVID-19 news encouraging, the family went from locked down to living life, overnight. "We weren't worrying about masks or sanitizing anymore," Martin said. "We were reacting to new information. Most people were not willing to do that. Even after the CDC said that COVID-19 had a ninety-nine percent survival rate."[61]

Signs of Approaching Finite Voltage

- **Flippant, cowboy attitude.** When a person believes they have faced all possible danger, and survived, they are liable to make a rookie mistake.

- **Short temper and lashing out in anger.** If someone is normally easy-going, but now they are snapping at people, they may be approaching burnout.
- **Lollygagging.** A sign often characterized by inattention to the task at hand, and looking at the ground more often than scanning the surroundings.

What to Do When You Are Burned Out

- **Take a break.** Even a simple, brief mental break, or a five-minute physical break, can help restore focus.
- **Acknowledge the burnout.** Cracked Boards and cut necktie mausoleums turn dangerous behaviors on their head by treating them as a rite of passage. These examples are a tacit acknowledgment that burnout has been achieved, and that absent a recharge, further mistakes are likely.
- **Do the next right thing.** Training exercises are designed to build instincts. Those instincts are supposed to kick in during times of stress. Do not get bored doing the right thing. Fall back on your training. Make the next right move.

Reaching or avoiding finite voltage is highly dependent on individual response to chaos events that can be modified by behavioral changes designed to pause thinking in the moment. But how does this affect future behavior?

ALL HANDS ON DECK: ROBERT TRAVIS

Living through perpetual chaos events changes the way we evaluate future safety threats. Robert Travis knows this firsthand. He was a sponsored professional snowboarder and a coach at the Camp of Champions in Whistler Blackcomb in British Columbia. Travis lived with impact and purpose. And then the twenty-two-year-old adrenaline addict split his tibia and fibula.

Pent-up during his recovery, Travis sought to make up for lost thrills. His interest was piqued by *Do You Have What It Takes?* advertisements seeking crew members for Alaskan fisheries. Crabbing was as notoriously dangerous as it was lucrative. "I didn't have a death wish," Travis said in a 2021 interview. "I was an elite athlete *and* I worked in concrete, both were grueling. I thought crabbing can't be harder than that."[62]

He contacted the Seattle-based recruiting firm in the TV ads and was hastily issued a plane ticket to Alaska. The only problem was his leg cast. "I cut it [the cast] off with an angle grinder," said Travis.[63]

He was assigned to one of the largest boats registered to compete in the crab season—a rugged, retrofitted 198-foot ex-buoy tender/icebreaker with an onboard processing plant and large cargo hold that allowed it to stay out a month before unloading at port.

Travis signed a contract and accepted almost certain maiming or death. Alternatively, if he survived, he would pocket $65,000 for four months' work. He was excited, and then hesitant.[64]

His first night on the ship was almost his last. Docked at Dutch Harbor, Travis woke at 4:00 a.m., packed his gear, clambered down the Jacob's ladder, and walked toward the airport. "This is stupid," he thought. "I've gotten in over my head."[65]

The first mate caught up to Travis and ordered him back to the boat. He refused. "You'll pay for your flight home," the mariner threatened.[66] Travis kept walking—and listening.

It obviously was not the first mate's only encounter with a jittery recruit. The officer adjusted his approach centering on the once-in-a-lifetime feat that forged men. After all, the vessel was undermanned, and they needed the greenhorn. The new approach worked.

Travis returned to the boat and began the first of two seasons fishing for crab. In 2003, he completed a 112-day contract and in 2007 returned for 119 days.[67] Describing his first season as an adventure, curiosity and newness were, however, distant feelings when he reported for his second season. He now had a family to support, and he understood what was in store for him.[68]

His first assignment in 2003 was that of processor working below the deck. In no time, a terrible injury to a deckhand resulted in Travis's promotion—and there he was, doing the most dangerous job on the boat with no training.[69]

The Bureau of Labor Statistics consistently rated fishing as the most hazardous occupation throughout much of the 1990s and 2000s. "In 2009, the rate of fatal injury for fishers and related fishing workers was 203.6 per 100,000 full-time equivalent workers, which is more than 50 times the all-worker rate of 3.5 per 100,000."[70]

Even in an insulated survival suit, death can come before help arrives. About 80 percent of crab fishery fatalities are from drowning.[71] Travis saw the searchlights of nearby boats trying to find and recover an overboard fisher. "We hauled up a guy in rain gear. He drowned. The Coast Guard came and got him."[72]

The Skipper's Buzzer

The skipper was in the wheelhouse three stories above the deck. His job was to drive the boat, to strategize fishing operations, and to protect the crew. He could position the boat to mitigate the jolt, dive, and roll from the towering swells.

Other times, he sounded the buzzer. "When you heard it, you grabbed onto whatever was nearest as fast as you could," said Travis.[73]

Although the buzzer might sound often during some shifts, it was impossible to predict exactly what was going to happen after it did. Sometimes refrigerator-sized slabs of ice careened over the gunwale, 800-pound crab cages broke loose, or 8-inch-deep ice water momentarily swirled on the deck, creating a riptide effect that swept crew members' feet from under them.[74]

It was not causal and it did not pattern. Positive recency meant nothing. If the boat responded in a specific way during the last five buzzers, then there was zero logic to support the proclamation "If *this* type of wave hits, then *this* will happen."

It was impossible to account for variables and there was never precision in the dynamic tempest of crab fishing. The baffles in the fuel tank and product tanks in the hold—would they fatigue or violently shift during a roll, transferring tons of force to one side of the boat? And ice. How thick was the ice on the superstructure and how was it distributed?

We Could Sink at Any Moment

Icing was a constant concern and demanded a generous cut of attention. The crew's job was dual: catch crab and fight the elements. "You would just finish your sixteen-hour shift, collapse in your bunk, and there would be an *all hands on deck* call," said Travis.[75]

Back on deck. If the boat iced over, it would lose buoyancy and sink. "We used baseball bats, pry bars, and ten-pound sledges to knock off the ice. It took hours, but if it built up too much and the boat rolled, it's bye, bye," recalled Travis.[76]

The job was mined with life-threatening obstacles that acted in inconceivable ways. On the stern, behind the wheelhouse, Travis was tossing garbage bags into an incinerator. The boat fell off a 40-foot wave. In an instant, he was 16 feet above the deck and falling.[77]

There is value in surviving narrow escapes. A fisher can be lured into a false sense of security that may prove fatal. That is the one skill you cannot accrue—safety. Improving safety is only possible with vigilance. And for almost everybody, such vigilance is impossible to maintain, especially in extended chaos situations.

All of My Bosses Are Dead

Four deck bosses. All killed by accidents on the boat; and unnumbered injuries and close calls. Travis remembers a shivering worker in the processing room warming his hands over a huge pot of scalding water used to flash-cook the crab.

"He was wearing layers of thick, insulated rubber gloves. To warm up, he dipped his hands into the water."[78] With its stabilizers removed from the conversion, the boat rolled 40 degrees when it fell into a trough. Travis did not recall hearing the buzzer.

"I watched the guy's eyes go wide. The water poured over the cuffs. He pulled out his hands and his face contorted in a horrible way. His fingers looked like bursting sausages."[79]

"You always had knives on you," said Travis. "A guy's hand got hooked on the automatic baiter. I cut him free. Another second and his arm would have been ripped clean from the shoulder. Those sorts of things happened *all* the time."[80]

Travis had brought 100 prescribed Tylenol-Codeine (T3) pills with him "just in case." Others discovered his stash and ate them like candy. Some of the crew leaned on narcotics and other [prohibited-on-the-boat] "medicine" to numb the pain or power them through shifts.[81]

What is resilience and what is luck? "You become very resilient, acquire mental tenacity, but how much of getting to the next day was skill or recognizing patterns or just luck?" questioned Travis.[82]

Once the ship left harbor, crew were cut off from the world beyond the boat. Cell phones did not work at sea. Travis received an annotated version of the month's news when the boat unloaded at port and the worn crew interlaced with busy land workers. As soon as the boat was tied off, the conveyors began offloading crab—an arduous process that took thirty-five to forty hours.

There were no escapes to taverns, restaurants, or hotels. At the time, ports had pay phones and these were sought after by crew—especially the guys with someone back home. "There would be thirty guys lined up at the telephone booth and you might get a minute or two to talk when it was your turn, 'Hey mom, I'm safe—talk to you in thirty days!'"[83]

The Final Days

The last days of the season were the most dangerous. "People got on each other's nerves even though they knew it was almost over," said Travis.[84] Everyone was exhausted, short-fused and ready-to-fight, wounded, and battling obscure infections known to those who fish for their living (figure 4.3).

There was also an earned hubris. Travis said, "You start to wonder if you are ever going to die—and a feeling that nothing can kill you. It was a dark place. That's when people became complacent and made lackadaisical errors. There are no inconsequential mistakes in that environment."[85]

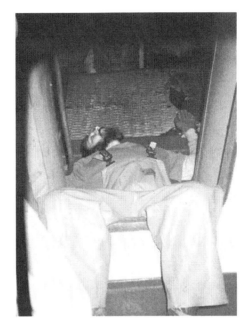

Figure 4.3 **Exhausted Deckhand Passed Out in a Doorway.** *Photo taken by Robert Travis on the boat, The Baranof, in November 2003. Credit Robert Travis.*

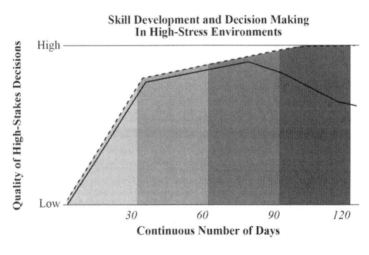

Figure 4.4 **Skill Development and Decision Making in High-Stress Environments.** *Credit David P. Perrodin and Aimee K. DiStefano.*

Crabbing seasons open in October, which is the month when the most fatal injuries happen to fishers. An argument could be made that some of these deaths are "rookie mistakes." But first-time errors do not account for the numbers during the final month of crabbing. February was the second most fatal month for fishers for the years 2003–2009.[86]

Although the crews' skills and competencies would increase over the course of the season, fatigue and resiliency collapse might have made their final days at sea nearly as dangerous as their first ones (figure 4.4).

Life after Dutch Harbor

Travis seldom talked about crabbing after he returned from Dutch Harbor. He found it difficult for others to understand his experiences—often insinuating he was a braggart. He savored moments to chat with sea fishermen who could relate to his stories, acknowledge the adversity, and empathize with his trauma.[87]

Having experienced never-ceasing chaos changed how Travis lived his life upon returning home. He evaluated daily situations for the probability of severe injury or death, and realized this as he instinctively positioned his family in the "most survivable" area of a ferry boat, which was a frequent means of transportation where he lived.

But this heightened situational awareness had a downside. Travis was benchmarking risks to what would be deemed life-threatening to a deckhand at sea. A danger threshold higher than that of the typical person. His calibration settings were iced over. This imbalance continues to affect him.

Travis admits that skewed judgment delayed his decision to abandon a large cement pour near Fort McMurray on May 2, 2016.[88] A mammoth forest fire raced toward him at 40 feet per minute. Authorities ordered 90,000 people to evacuate. Travis was aware of the situation and overestimated his ability to impose order during chaos. He believed that he would find an egress, even in the final seconds.

There was no skipper to sound the buzzer. As luck would have it, Travis's wife was looking out for him. She convinced Travis to rush to a safer area.

The Fort McMurray, Alberta wildfire was dubbed "the beast" for its merciless unpredictability. "The Insurance Bureau of Canada pegged the Fort McMurray fire as the costliest insured natural disaster in Canadian history."[89]

He was not allowed back to the area until June 15. The entire worksite was incinerated.

After the fire, Travis became an entrepreneur. Applying what he learned from his experiences on the storm-tossed Bering Sea, he co-founded a company that designs and builds fast-deployment urban life rafts to help people survive floods in residential areas.

Takeaways from Robert Travis

- **Do Not be Lulled by Positive Recency.** If a flipped coin lands on its head a dozen times in a row, the thirteenth flip still only has a probability of 50 percent heads or 50 percent tails.
- **Be Alert for Signs of Gradual Decline into Disorder.** A persistent threat to a Bering Sea fisher was that the boat would become layered with ice, lose buoyancy, and sink. The natural decay of structures proceeds so slowly that we seldom notice the changes as they happen.
- **Decision-Making Will Crest and Then Fall.** Anticipate fatigue in decision-making around sixty days into a high-stress environment. Although skills continue to increase, there is not a corresponding decrease in the danger of the task.

CIVILIAN MORALE DURING UNCERTAIN TIMES

Militaries fight wars, but entire nations go to war. Never is the consent of the governed more important than in wartime.

Most of the public will never be called to fight, even in the case of a draft. But all have a role to play. Someone has to grow the food war fighters eat, write the letters they read, buy the bonds that fund the war, and see to the care of the wounded soldier or their family. The government cannot do it all. Besides, it is too busy fighting a war. Those roles must be not only filled, but embraced.

Much like the sitcom spouse who wants their partner to *want* to do the dishes, propaganda directed at civilians tries to nudge them into identifying a patriotism of their own. A farmer's contribution to the war looks different from a banker's which looks different from an elementary school class writing letters to the hometown warrior on the front lines. Governments want and need them all and cannot do much of that itself.

In the sections ahead, we will survey some of the most important propaganda campaigns in history. Two of the most fascinating took place during World War I, and show how propaganda took different forms on opposite sides of the Atlantic Ocean.

In the Habsburg Empire, modern-day Austria, civilians donating to a relief fund for warriors earned the right to hammer a nail into a wooden statue in the town square. With each gift and each nail, the Iron Soldier transformed, right before the public's eyes.

And in America, an army of Four-Minute Men offered pro-war talking points in brief speeches, a direct line from President Woodrow Wilson's desk to a nation's ears. Whether the crown or a democracy, governments understand the importance of high civilian spirits in a time of sacrifice. Let us take a look at how they lift those spirits.

Hammering the *Wehrmann in Eisen*

Every war is fought on two fronts: the battlefield and the dinner table. Since 1914, the start of World War I, "war has increasingly involved the nation as a whole—the man, woman and child behind the lines, as well as the soldier at the front," noted a post-World War II U.S. Air Force research paper on civilian morale.[90]

Battlefield morale can mean the difference between winning and losing the battle. And a battle could mean the difference between winning and losing the war. Keeping the men who fight their nation's battles in the mood and spirit to do so is understood to be a matter of literal national security.

But civilian morale matters, too. The people at the dinner table send their sons, husbands, and brothers off to war. Some will never return. And some will never be whole again. Wars are fought in the public's name, and with its money. If war is hell, as the saying goes, the heat had better be worth it.

World War I was a disaster for Europe. The Austro-Hungarian Empire suffered some of the continent's deepest losses. The story of one of Europe's last royal dynasties, the Habsburg Empire, reveals the truth of finite voltage: no matter how novel or inclusive, or how propagandistic and rosy morale campaigns are when they start, reality sets in eventually.

In 1915, a wooden statue of a soldier was erected in a town square in Vienna. A story on *Atlas Obscura* explained: "For a small donation, members of the public could help sheath the knight in nail head armor, one nail at a time. The funds raised . . . went to underwrite the costs of supporting the widows and orphans of World War I."[91]

Some 500,000 nails were hammered into the wooden statue, called the *Wehrmann in Eisen*. From German, that translates to "Iron Soldier." Just as war hardens the men who fight it, each donation and each hammered-in nail transformed the soldier from wood to iron.

The inscription under the statue reads: "Iron man of Vienna commemorates the time when suffering brought by war was as great as love and charity!"[92] Only in the sword the Iron Soldier carries do its modest wood beginnings still show through.

That the Iron Soldier is not steeled, completely, despite all the donations and despite all the hammering, takes on a symbolic meaning: Both the men who fight wars and the civilians who support them are only human. Everybody has limits.

The physical, public, and communal nature of the Iron Soldier allowed people who could not participate on the front lines of battle—such as women, children, and the elderly—still to make a contribution. Donors got their name in the donation book. People could be seen hammering nails and supporting the war.

There is doing the right thing, and then there is being seen doing the right thing. The Iron Soldier allowed donors to do both.

The Iron Soldier was novel and communal, at first. But "after a few years the novelty of the Wehrmann would wear thin," according to *The International Encyclopedia of the First World War*.[93] Marketing campaigns, no matter how communal, do not overcome harsh reality. Not when the harsh reality goes on seemingly without end.

It was the "few years" that was the problem. Any one strategy will yield diminishing returns over time. Whether it was the Iron Soldier or war bonds, eventually the reality of the war, and its duration, burned out even the most patriotic.

A jolt of patriotic fervor, at the outset of war, is to be expected. That is when people's resistance to voltage is the highest because it has not yet been tested. The civilian populace is still fresh. They have not suffered losses yet.

But when the war dragged on for years and years—the World War I Armistice was not called until November 11, 1918, three years after the wooden soldier was rolled to Vienna—the hammering of the 500,000th nail takes on a different, and lesser, meaning than the 5,000th.

After a certain point, all of it was about a war whose costs were increasingly high, and whose benefit was tough to see.

In the end, Austria-Hungary lost 1.5 million soldiers in the war, another half-million civilians, and the Habsburg family, royalty since 1273, was demoted to mere nobility. Not even a centuries-old empire could sustain the weight of "the war to end war."

Finite voltage applies to royals and commoners both.

The Four-Minute Men

In 1917, during World War I, President Woodrow Wilson deployed some 75,000 "Four-Minute Men" to speak in favor of the war effort in their communities. Essentially a volunteer civilian-morale army, the Four-Minute Men delivered propaganda with a personal touch.

The effort was orchestrated by Wilson's Committee on Public Information, a predecessor to the Committee for National Morale. Both efforts were meant to influence Americans to partake in the world war of their time.

Bulletins were sent to speakers offering helpful hints. Brevity was important. "There is no time for a single wasted word," instructed the inaugural bulletin, published May 22, 1917.[94] "Divide your speech carefully into certain divisions, say 15 seconds for final appeal; 45 seconds to describe the bond; 15 seconds for opening words."[95] The spoken word from a polished rhetorician was a premium communication during a time when 6 percent of people in America fourteen years old and older were illiterate (unable to read or write in *any* language).[96]

A September 1917 story in *The Topeka Daily Capital* hailed the Four-Minute Men of Kansas as "the biggest army ever organized in the state."[97]

"Women will not be barred from service if they can stand up and preach patriotism from their shoulder," the front-page story reads. "But it's got to be the real article, for the 'Four-Minute Men' will not be recruited from the sob squad."[98]

Four-Minute Men, and women, would give their speeches in "every movie house in the state," often before or between a showing of newsreels. To ensure this, the Wilson Administration made sure the Kansas censor board turned over a list of all the movie houses.

"The owners of these movie houses will be asked to sandwich in a speech by a local spellbinder between reels at every entertainment, afternoon and evening," the story read.[99] The Four-Minute Men delivered messages of propaganda in a distinctly personal manner. In Britain, however, the message was delivered by poster board.

Which Pain Will You Choose for Yourself?

Whether or not fighting in World War I was a fit for your life plan was beside the point. Propaganda was designed to train the individual to uplift other interests above his own. Everywhere a young man went, he could be expected to see his older self on a poster. The daughter he does not yet have, but will, is sitting on his lap with a large book open in her hand.

She looks beseechingly at her father. But it is clear further admiration might be dependent on the answer to her question: "Daddy, what did you do in the Great War?" Dad, wearing a three-piece suit, looks wistfully into the distance.

We never know his answer, but the pained expression on his face could only come from one of two places: remembering the horrors of the war he fought, or regret that he stayed home when others fought. Which pain will you choose for yourself, young man? Every young man in Britain was made to face that question every time he saw a propaganda poster.

It worked. In one year, from August 1914 to September 1915, more than two million men signed up to fight under the Union Jack.[100] The National War Savings Committee, organized by Lord Robert Kindersley, sought investments in war bonds from four million Brits to finance the war effort.

The first government bond in Britain was issued by Britain in 1693 to fund a war against France.[101] By World War I, the war bond was a British tradition hundreds of years in the making. Just as men of war-fighting age were propagandized to fight, women and men too old to fight were encouraged to buy bonds. Neighbors formed savings groups in their neighborhoods.

While the Austrians hammered half-a-million nails into their Iron Soldier during World War I and the Four-Minute Men delivered their briefings, the British bought 432 million pounds of war bonds. Nearly half-a-billion.[102] In the years following World War I, the means of delivering propaganda began to change, under influence by changing technology.

ROOSEVELT'S FIRESIDE CHATS—
THE MEDIUM IS THE MAGIC

Franklin Delano Roosevelt's presidency stands out not only for its duration but also the challenges he and America faced together from 1933 to 1945, from the Great Depression to World War II. The enormity of those two challenges, but especially the Depression, which welcomed FDR to office, forced him to the radio airwaves, early and often, in his now famous "fireside chats."

The fireside chat was the creation of a White House aide. The idea was that beaming the president's words, live, from his house to yours, unfiltered by time or editors, would allow unprecedented intimacy between the president and the public. "To many, the Great Depression confirmed what they had suspected all along: individuals no longer mattered in the new economic order."[103]

Roosevelt was eager to change that impression. By the time he was inaugurated, there had been a months-long "run on the banks," wherein people were liquidating their accounts into cash, burning through banks' holdings and causing many to collapse. As indicators of the national economy go, these were bad ones. They were not just warning signs. This action was trouble itself.

The first fireside chat went out live just eight days after FDR's inauguration, on March 12, 1933. "I want to talk for a few minutes with the people of the United States about banking," he said at the start of the inaugural chat.[104]

The fireside chats were "the first media events—live, pre-planned, extraordinary broadcasts that riveted the attention of the nation—in American history," writes history professor David Ryfe.[105] "Roosevelt often used the 'you' form," Ryfe continues "throughout the chats, he is concerned to 'tell you,' 'interest you,' 'make it clear to you,' and 'make you understand.'"[106] It was as if the president were speaking directly to each individual.

Despite the fact that millions of people could be listening at any moment, all of them were doing so in intimate spaces, in their cars or their homes. This intimacy was unlike every other political speech in history. And it was the medium, radio, that made the difference.

In decades of old, to hear a politician give a speech, people gathered at train stations. After being elected president in 1860, Abraham Lincoln gave his farewell to Illinois at the train station in Springfield on February 11, 1861, before getting onboard, en route to Washington, D.C. (In Lincoln's and in Roosevelt's time, presidents were inaugurated in March.) "I now leave, not knowing when or whether I ever may return," Lincoln said, words which proved prophetic.[107]

Before the advent of radio, the trend was "stump" speeches where the speaker literally stood on a sawed-off tree trunk while the crowd gathered around to listen. FDR's radio addresses took political speech away from the exclusive province of whistle stops and tree stumps and moved it into the living room.

People no longer had to venture physically into the town square to hear what was being said there. A man whose physical disabilities would have prevented him from giving traditional stump speeches turned tradition on its head by using the radio and reaching people where they were.

Radio allowed a person to be a citizen in the comfort of their own home. It would take a whole lot of tree stumps to match the audience of even one fireside chat. Creativity and technology helped FDR turn his physical limitation into unprecedented reach.

The newness of it all—a new president using a new medium to reach out in a new way—was compelling. Newspapers were in their final stand on the mountaintop. Radio gained ground by the day, as live broadcasts, especially of the president's remarks, carried more urgency than the written word. The newspaper was old by the time it reached you. It had been touched by many hands. It could be read, or put aside, at any time.

But people had to plan to catch a radio appearance. For all they knew then, they would never have the chance to hear it again. However, in recent years, some have claimed that the fireside chats were not *really* that intimate. Proof offered for this claim lies in that FDR did not speak the language of the common man, did not share his innermost thoughts, and used the fireside chats for name-calling opponents.[108]

"Why . . . has the fire in the fireside chats been overlooked?" author Elvin T. Lim asks. He argues that the "illusion of intimacy" of the fireside chats does not meet any definition of that word. Besides that, Lim notes, the fireplace in the White House's Diplomatic Reception Room, where the addresses were given, was never even used.[109] But that analysis isolates the message from the medium, when the two are indivisible.

Even an in-depth analysis of FDR's word choices and speech topics ignores the inherent intimacy and novelty of live speeches at that time. What could be *more* intimate, after all, than learning what the president of the United States is thinking, at the same time the rest of the world does?

Regardless of what words the president was using, you were hearing them simultaneously with the Speaker of the House, the Queen of England, or anyone else who might be listening. Roosevelt's use of the radio medium is so well-regarded that it became a tradition, which goes on to this day as the sitting president's weekly radio address. Donald Trump briefly ended the tradition when he moved to social media communications but Joe Biden brought it back.[110]

That homage, long-standing and ongoing, is an acknowledgment that "today's presidents . . . live in the shadow of [FDR's] oratorical genius."[111] But codifying novelty into tradition also ignores the importance of medium to the message. Radio was new when FDR used it. It became outmoded when TV became widespread, and then cable. It is archaic in the Internet age. A president using radio, at this late date, is drinking from the well FDR dug almost ninety years ago.

The modern-day equivalent, a president using a relatively new medium to spread influence in a new way, would be a president using TikTok videos to reach young people. But radio was only part of the FDR magic. He did not just use his bully pulpit to talk at people. He showed an interest in their lives. He encouraged people to write letters and then talked about the letters he received.

People were flattered that their president cared enough to ask. Here was the president of the United States, starting every radio speech with "my friends," talking honestly about the challenges they face, and even asking to hear about them.

Whereas FDR's predecessor, Herbert Hoover, received about 800 letters a day—which was 800 more than he asked for—FDR got 8,000 per day. "Americans responded to FDR's radio talks with an unprecedented tide of mail," according to a 2014 analysis. "A fireside chat could generate some 450,000 letters, cards and telegrams."[112]

The reactions themselves varied wildly. On October 1, 1934, Melvin Chisum from Philadelphia, a self-described "red hot, jet-black Democrat," and field secretary of the National Negro Press Association, wrote to the president: "You know what your government is doing. You know how to explain it. You know where you are heading and you are on your way."[113]

That same day, Hugh Colliton Jr., of Wayland, Massachusetts, cited the same speech Chisum did as "a display of mental incompetency," adding that "a small-time politician could really have done better."[114]

In his weekly presidential radio addresses, Jimmy Carter tried to restore that two-way connection between president and public by taking calls from listeners. It was not the same. Letters scale up in a way calls do not. Even an ambitious effort to hear people out might take only ten calls in one hour.

Many people held warm memories of writing to the White House because FDR asked them to do so. Not so much the callers to Jimmy Carter's radio hour. Maybe the president would read your letter himself. Maybe he would even read it on the air. Maybe a staffer would read it on orders of the president. But even if nothing came of it, it was the thought that counted.

Using that powerful feeling of personal connection, FDR had honed his fireside chat skills during the Great Depression. World War II pushed him to use those skills to raise the morale of a nation once again.

COMMITTEE FOR NATIONAL MORALE

America had been on the road to World War II for months by the time the Japanese attacked Pearl Harbor in December 1941. Now America was on the road to victory. It had to be. America was the "last, best hope of Earth."[115]

Months before the attack, during a fireside chat, President Roosevelt declared an "unlimited national emergency" owing to the war.[116] Still, America sat on the sideline. As long as it could. But Pearl Harbor changed everything.

Punctured, for decades—before it went away forever on 9/11—was the myth that America's two oceans and friendly neighbors exempted it from outside attack. America did not want war, but war wanted America.

Propaganda, for Democracy's Sake

In July 1940, after World War II had begun, but before America joined the fight, the Committee for National Morale was formed as an advisory group to President Roosevelt. The Committee was an assemblage of about sixty thought leaders brought together to study morale in America and the propaganda tactics of the Axis Powers, and to respond with a uniquely American form of propaganda, one that would urge people together rather than forcing them apart, as the Nazis did.

The Committee was not formed to beat the drums for war, exactly, but to help form the kind of "democratic personality" that would make Americans better disposed to play a role in a war, if it were to happen. The Committee operated from a belief that "in the present crisis . . . morale will probably be the decisive factor and that the United States must employ her tremendous morale resources to the fullest extent for a long time to come."[117]

The approach to producing American propaganda incorporated democratic ideals in novel ways. "Policymakers perceived their job as more than keeping tabs on what Americans were thinking and feeling; they had to skillfully engineer the appropriate U.S. outlook," Ellen Herman wrote.[118] Six months after Pearl Harbor, in May 1942, the U.S. government and the world of high art collaborated to produce an immersive art installation that would change one heart and mind at a time.

Road to Victory

"Road to Victory: A Procession of Photographs of a Nation at War," had a six-month run at New York's Museum of Modern Art, from May to October 1942. "It is by no means a photography exhibition in the ordinary sense but one of the most powerful propaganda efforts yet attempted," read the press release announcing the exhibit.[119]

Fred Turner, an author and communications professor at Stanford University, described *Road to Victory* as an "extremely successful propaganda exhibition," and an example of what he calls a "democratic surround," during a guest appearance on the Center for Humane Technology's *The Undivided Attention Podcast*.[120]

Surrounds are "environments that surround people with images," said Turner, author of *The Democratic Surround: Multimedia and American Liberalism from World War II to the Psychedelic Sixties*.[121]

Road to Victory offered "that vision of a world in which you could see yourself among others unlike you, and yet perceive yourself as collectively part of a larger mission to build a better world. And to resist massification, and to resist fascism," Turner said.[122] "To resist bigotry of the antisemitic kind that was clearly driving fascism in Germany. That was a beautiful thing, and people responded to it."[123] Respond they did. In eight weeks, about 80,000 guests came through, and photos of displays were widely disseminated in newspapers around America.

Tristan Harris, host of *The Undivided Attention Podcast*, called the Committee's work "a democratic propaganda," set forth to influence people—as propaganda does—but not in the dehumanizing way it was done in Nazi Germany.[124] The idea was not that propaganda is different when America does it, but that America does propaganda differently. And better.

Turner quotes psychologist Abraham Maslow, creator of the hierarchy of human needs, on what sets the democratic personality apart from the fascism of the Axis world: "The democratic person tends to respect other human beings in a very basic fashion as different from each other, rather than better or worse here. . . . People are human beings and therefore unique and respect worthy."[125]

The inherent intricacy was "[w]hat they had to produce in their own minds was [that] American unity that was not at the same time an authoritarian style of unity," according to Turner.[126]

The highest levels of American arts and letters collaborated on *Road to Victory*. Herbert Bayer designed the exhibit, which required shifting the movable interior walls of the museum's second floor. Carl Sandburg, a poet and historian fresh off winning a Pulitzer for his 1940 biography of President Abraham Lincoln, smithed the words. His brother-in-law, Lieutenant Commander Edward Steichen, a photographer with the U.S. Naval Reserves, shot some of the photos and oversaw the installation.[127]

The exhibit showed off "not only its fighting men but the country's resources and its people—farmers, workers, housewives, mothers, fathers, children—will be shown in mural-size enlargements," the announcement read.[128]

Road to Victory depicted Americans as black and white, and as rural, urban, and suburban. It showed them at home, at war, at work, and at play. "Country boys, big city lads, hometown fellers, they're in the Army now," read one of Sandburg's captions.[129] Below it, two of those lads and fellers cross a bridge, rifle bayonets drawn.

One picture shows a pair of Connecticut tobacco farmers enjoying a light moment away from the fields. As the man cinches his waist and looks off into the distance, his wife lets out a hearty laugh. Sandburg's caption: "The earth is alive. The land laughs. The people laugh. And the fat of the land is here."[130]

In those days, propaganda came clearly labeled. For the *Road to Victory* exhibit, the words were written by a Pulitzer winner, and the photographs were chosen to tug at the heartstrings. But you knew who was doing the tugging: Uncle Sam. And you knew why: to get all 135 million Americans to take on a role, some role, in an all-encompassing war effort.

The End of Opt-In Propaganda

Eighty years after *Road to Victory*, the tools of propaganda are not as clearly labeled, and the delivery mechanisms have changed. The word itself, *propaganda*, was still in regular use back in the 1940s. It was still a neutral term then, a tactic rather than the four-letter word it became. Over the course of World War II, propaganda obtained a negative connotation as something only the Nazis would do. Or those of their ilk.

That stigma is likely why people engage now in propaganda without using the word. In the 2020s, we are all propagandized now. All day. On our TVs, on our computers, and on our phones.

Back during the two world wars, American propaganda was an opt-in experience. You had to be in the church when the Four-Minute Man was talking. You would have to walk into the theater where the propaganda film was playing.

In 1942, someone who wanted to walk the *Road to Victory* had to be in New York, go to the museum, pay an entry fee, and climb to the second floor. Immersion required real effort.

In the 2020s, all you need to do is pull your phone out of your pocket. Who is pulling the strings? What do they want from you? The answers to those questions depend on the medium, the messenger, and the moment. Harris, a design ethicist, argues that the "surrounds" of our time are our smartphones. He questions how "democratic" they are, and how healthful. "Essentially the smartphones, Facebook, newsfeeds, Instagram, TikTok, YouTube, are the new democratic surrounds," Harris said.[131]

The danger is that our phones are "polarizing surrounds" or "outrage surrounds" or "conspiracy surrounds," and we do not even know it, Harris said.[132] We come into contact with propaganda very differently today than people did a century ago. Information is moving faster than humans have ever experienced.

Propaganda is no longer something people opt into. They can hardly opt out, even if they want to do so. We do not have to walk into an immersive art experience, watch newsreels, or even put on a virtual reality headset to be propagandized these days. A fusillade of ideas rains down upon us every time we unlock our phones.

Keys to Managing Civilian Morale

- **Roles boost morale.** Developing roles for citizens is nothing new, exemplified in World War I times by the creation of the Four-Minute Men. During the COVID-19 pandemic, local governments in America offered web portals where people could report neighbors hosting "too many" guests. If staying home meant staying safe, people who left home were being unsafe, many believed. People who might otherwise be angered at social restrictions found purpose in aiding the government's enforcement of those restrictions.[133]
- **Winning the home front takes a village.** Shows of solidarity such as the Iron Soldier allowed an entire community to signal their support for the men fighting in their defense. People could give to the war effort and be seen as giving.
- **Propaganda, communicated early and frequently, moves the consumer to Point B. The risk of over-communicating is less important than leaving the field open to catastrophic rumors.** Whether it is Four-Minute Men speaking in theaters, FDR giving fireside chats via radio, or an art installation like *Road to Victory*, propaganda is offered to inspire action.

We all burn out eventually. Tactics lose their novelty over the long run. Human capacity for sacrifice is not unlimited. People, and even empires, such as the Habsburgs in Europe, reach their end eventually. However, when a whole population reaches finite voltage, a chaos event can sometimes be extended.

DR. DAVID MAYS—POPULATION-LEVEL FINITE VOLTAGE AND POLITICS PROLONGED A PANDEMIC

It is a taboo thought. But in the early days of the COVID-19 pandemic, there was something electric and palpable about the sense of change. It was a time unlike any other.

"At first, everything's fun for a lot of people," said Dr. David Mays, M.D., Ph. D., a Wisconsin-based forensic psychiatrist, in April 2021 during a private interview about the events of a year prior.[134]

"No one says that, but that's actually what we're feeling: 'We have to hunker down, I don't have to go to work anymore.' And it'll be this fun, 'we're being snowed-in experience,'" Dr. Mays said.[135]

Dr. Mays, who has written over a dozen research publications, presented nearly 700 academic workshops since 2005, and received at least ten awards in his field, currently serves as Clinical Adjunct Assistant Professor in the Department of Psychiatry at the University of Wisconsin.

With more than thirty years of experience treating patients and researching mental illness, personality disorders, and suicide in environments such as prisons and group homes, Dr. Mays has an uncommon vantage on finite voltage in group settings. COVID-19 was a unique test of the finite voltage of the general public, unlike in its scale from even world wars of the past.

Dr. Mays believes there was a heightened sense of possibility in those early days, when the newness of the virus was fresh. People were at home, and watching daily government press conferences. From those lecterns, governors and mayors and even the president would issue orders affecting their livelihood at work and their ability to move about freely.

If the need for three weeks of stay-at-home sacrifice had been laid out early on, and enforced tightly, Dr. Mays postulates that the pandemic might have lasted several weeks, instead of stretching out more than a year.[136]

"This Is an Emergency"

As COVID-19 spread from state to state, and state governors issued stay-at-home orders, the difference between 2020 and life before the virus could not have been starker.

Overnight, there were few cars on the road, and few places to go other than the grocery store. The drive-thru lines at fast-food restaurants such as McDonald's were wrapped around the block. Toilet paper was hard to find, and bleach wipes nearly impossible. For once, the panic seemed to justify the panic-buying.

Dr. Mays feels those changes were not enough. With a strict, widely accepted lockdown, the virus would have probably become manageable in less than a month. But the political divide made that sacrifice too big an ask, in some quarters. Dr. Mays believes that politics of selfishness and denial won out, and in so doing, made the pandemic longer-lasting and more hurtful than it needed to be.[137]

"In three weeks, this virus is gone in a quarantined, controlled population," Dr. Mays said, reflecting his thoughts early in the pandemic. "If it's not being spread, and other people aren't getting it and bringing it in, it's going to be gone."[138]

The proper messaging, according to Dr. Mays, would have been: "This is an emergency. We're giving you a couple of days, then we're shutting everything down. No more work, no businesses, no banks, no buses, nothing. Go home."[139]

"There was kind of an exciting urgency at the time and I think most people felt that," Dr. Mays said. "We could do that for three weeks. But we couldn't do that for a year and a half."[140]

The Crisis of a Lifetime

For people who felt that history had evaded them, and they were cursed to just living an ordinary life, the pandemic was the kind of event that fills history books. But with the arrival of a once-in-a-century pandemic, history was no longer the exclusive terrain of those people in *Time-Life* magazines of old. For at least fifteen months, life and history were interchangeable.

But the excitement of the early days soon faded. In America, each state formed its own plan to fight the virus. COVID-19 infection numbers and the conditions of life varied widely both from state to state and from county to county. Permissible activities were tied to confusing criteria and the ineffectiveness resembled the ill-fated five color-coded levels of the terrorist threat system implemented by Homeland Security following the 9/11 attacks. Is today Level Orange or Level Yellow? What are the differences?

"At about three months, people said, 'I don't want to do this anymore,'" Dr. Mays observed.[141] The population's collectively frayed nerves were sparking like downed power lines. Pressure pushed many to their finite voltage.

Masks, especially, became a flashpoint of controversy. They should not have. Dr. Mays is a clinical professor at the University of Wisconsin in Madison. Despite its status as the capital city, within Wisconsin, Madison is viewed as a liberal college town, like Ann Arbor is in Michigan or Austin is in Texas. Dr. Mays said that when he would speak to statewide groups, he was urged to avoid mention of masks, lest he be written off as an out-of-touch Madisonian.

"This is in the midst of the worst epidemic, and there is no reason not to wear a mask, other than its inconvenience," Dr. Mays said. "That was political. That was a response to the collapse of resilience."[142]

As time went on, cracks in the stay-home-and-stay-safe consensus grew in almost every state. Masks were controversial in some states, such as Texas, from the beginning. Sometimes, as in Michigan, the battle lines were drawn by party, with Republicans taking Governor Gretchen Whitmer, a Democrat, to court to have her executive orders thrown out.[143] And other times, in one-party-led states such as New York, it was lawmakers clawing back power from the then-chief executive Governor Andrew Cuomo.[144]

Whether the fault lines were drawn between parties or branches of government, it was clear that America's political leaders were not "all in it together." After finite voltage burned out, politics was a power game again. Just like in the before-times.

Trust Issues

The pandemic did not last the three weeks Dr. Mays had hoped.

On May 13, 2021, the Centers for Disease Control and Prevention said vaccinated people could stop wearing masks indoors or out. The goal for "herd immunity," or 70 percent of adults immunized, had not nearly been achieved. Deaths were still in the double-digits daily in most states, and triple-digits nationwide.[145] The rolling seven-day death toll was 622 according to *The New York Times* Data Tracker.[146]

So what changed?

Dr. Mays believes that the judgment came too early, and without basis. The population may have reached finite voltage on COVID-19, but Dr. Mays is holding strong to his mask. In late May 2021, about two weeks after the CDC order, he admitted: "I have a post-COVID-19 anxiety about not wearing a mask."[147]

"It's hard to not wear a mask," Dr. Mays continued. "I like being behind the mask and feeling that I was somehow safe. I have some lingering anxiety about being in the general public."[148] The politicization of the virus and the government's seemingly random decision to lift the mask mandate leaves Dr. Mays low on trust when it comes to government orders and proclamations of safety.

Overnight, fellow shoppers were unmasked at the grocery store. Some even offered their hands for handshakes. Regardless of what daily death and case tolls indicated, in the minds of most Americans, the ability to remove masks meant the pandemic was over.

Dr. Mays questions that view and is disturbed at its endorsement by the same institutions urging caution just a year prior. "What changed overnight? The COVID-19 numbers were still high. COVID-19 was still around," Dr. Mays said in the May 2021 interview. "It felt like the machinery of government and business were going to push forward regardless of the data."[149]

"I have very little confidence in any sort of government at this point," Dr. Mays lamented. "I don't trust what their agenda is."[150] Ironically, that same sentiment is shared by those who opposed mask mandates all along. To avoid this generalized loss of trust, could messaging about the pandemic have been handled differently?

THE EVENT 201 PANDEMIC EXERCISE

On October 18, 2019, the Johns Hopkins Center for Health Security in partnership with the World Economic Forum and the Bill and Melinda Gates Foundation hosted Event 201, a high-level global pandemic exercise held in New York City.[151] The purpose of the activity was to strengthen the shared response by governments and businesses to a global pandemic.

Event 201 was proactive and tactical, and also narrow and incomplete. It was a bit like planning for a meteor impact by tuning the space laser weapons as you don headphones to drown out the screams of seven billion humans. The population was an afterthought.

The by-invitation-only event's "players" consisted of fifteen prominent individuals from global business, government, and public health. Rostering the brain trust were Dr. Lotaya D. Abbott, Senior Director of Global Occupational Health Services for Marriott International, Dr. Stephen C. Redd, Deputy Director for Public Health Service and Implementation Science at the Centers for Disease Control and Prevention (CDC), and Adrian Thomas, Vice President Global Public Health at Johnson & Johnson.[152]

A hefty line-up of right-handed batters, indeed. A behavioral scientist, a Daniel Kahneman-type, might have balanced the quantitative leanings of the specialists. Somebody who would stand on the qualitative side of the plate.

Beyond the conference room in The Big Apple was a world that had not endured a globe-hopping virus for a century. The simulation had been planned and held months before the first report of coronavirus disease in Wuhan, China in December 2019.[153]

But in October 2019, American newscasts wrapped up coverage of Hurricane Dorian's dismantling of the Bahamas and thrashing of America's Atlantic basin. The Event 201 tabletop exercise did not flag the public's attention. In fact, most news about it originated from its own press releases.

Although this activity has a curious placement on the COVID-19 timeline, its facilitators were attentive to public transparency. When COVID-19 went online, Event 201 was not taken offline. The event's recommendations, neatly curated, were available to the public from its website (including full-length videos the group posted to YouTube).[154]

Yet, where was the Event 201 all-star team at the onset of, or at any time during, the COVID-19 pandemic? To inform the pandemic scenario, Center for Health Security scholars had researched CAPS (Coronavirus Acute Pulmonary Syndrome): The Pathogen and Clinical Syndrome, Communication in a Pandemic, Finance in a Pandemic, and Medical Countermeasures.[155]

It is logical, at face value, that these fifteen informed experts would have been heavily leaned upon, even showcased, by world governments both to convey competent forethought and boost the public morale: here are your heroes!

Whether by oversight or by intention, keeping these experts off the world stage was a major blunder by national governments. And either way, the forensic optics underscores this colossal misstep. The collective group should have been present behind the White House podium as *the* face of the COVID-19 task force in March 2020. It made sense.

The Event 201 recommendations document begins with, "The next severe pandemic will not only cause great illness and loss of life but could also trigger major cascading economic and societal consequences that could contribute greatly to global impact and suffering."[156] The four-page report then breaks into seven points about public-private cooperation for pandemic preparedness and response.

Sections 1 through 6 are centered on international collaboration and managing assets. In fact, the recommendations, although broad, were calibrated with reasonable tolerance to what would unfold in 2020—with one glaring omission.

Section 7 landed closest to a population-level civilian morale campaign by championing reliable public messaging and amplifying credible information.[157] But it fell short of prioritizing population morale and its treatment. In fact, the words "morale," "mental health," "depression," "attitude," or "psychology" do not appear in the recommendations document.

By hyper-focusing on systems, the civilians went out of focus. This omission was a lost opportunity because a start-of-pandemic reincarnation of a Committee for National Morale-esque ensemble would have set a cornerstone of optimism.

HOME FRONT MORALE IN 2020— FITNESS AND FORTITUDE

The U.S. government squandered an opportunity to launch decisively a tone-setting civilian morale program at the onset of the COVID-19 pandemic. Instead of executive leadership and actionable guidance, confined Americans were spinning in their own circles, dabbling in DIY mask-making, and figuring out which celebrity had the best technique for disinfecting phones.

It was an uncoordinated carnival of "this might help" ring tosses that made it appear that we had no counter punch to adversity. By contrast, the American government had a different, and better, approach to maintaining high civilian morale at the outset of World War II.

In the nascent days of the COVID-19 pandemic, Americans scoured the waves, eager to partake in a *Road to Victory*-type event that would coalesce them into a continuous unified force. What was something that everyone could participate in? A food drive? That will not work during a pandemic when people are being told that they will be safer at home. But thinking more about food—How about nutrition? How about fitness?

Dr. Anthony Fauci was on board. He recommended getting enough sleep, maintaining a healthy diet, and avoiding or alleviating stress as the most potent ways to keep your immune system strong.

In an interview with *Business Insider*, the seventy-nine-year-old head of the National Institute of Allergy and Infectious Diseases, shared "I go for my exercise—a three- to four-mile power walk at night with my wife."[158]

Like the Faucis, Americans needed to get moving, get fit, and become a harder target for COVID-19. #FitnessFortitude. The correlation between fitness and nutrition increasing the immune system is proven—to the point it is an axiom.

We know fitness and nutrition are good for everyone, for all living creatures. Not just good for the body, but good for the mind. The statement, "fatigue makes cowards of us all" has been attributed to both General George Patton and Green Bay Packers coach Vince Lombardi. Without proper exercise and fuel, both the body and mind are more easily susceptible to fatigue.

The COVID-19 fitness research was falling into place, too. In a July 2020 study published in the *Journal of Clinical and Experimental Medicine*, researchers wrote,

> The practice of physical activities strengthens the immune system, suggesting a benefit in the response to viral communicable diseases. Thus, regular practice of adequate intensity is suggested as an auxiliary tool in strengthening and preparing the immune system for COVID-19.[159]

If only there were a national civilian fitness vessel, one that could be hurried into drydock, primed, painted, and sent back to duty.

In 2015, the U.S. Army introduced the Army Civilian Fitness Program. "The Army Civilian Fitness Program is designed to encourage civilian employees to improve their health and fitness through formal physical exercise training and other wellness activities."[160]

Fitness does not only improve physical shape. According to the Comprehensive Soldier Fitness website, the Army Civilian Fitness Program has been shown to help boost morale, improve health and fitness, and increase productivity in the workplace.[161]

And, fitness is inclusive. It was the perfect population-level campaign to launch early in March 2020.

According to professional strength trainer Drew Baye, "If you can contract your muscles voluntarily, you can exercise."[162] Baye has trained paraplegics, hemiplegics, people with joint and spine problems, and individuals with serious birth defects affecting limb development.

You can become fit without leaving the house. Baye said, "It doesn't have to be a barbell, dumbbell, cable, or machine. Something as simple as a strap or yoga block or household structure you can contract against can be used to exercise effectively."[163]

The Army's fitness program should have been scaled to engage the national population level through website and app-based applications.

Tweak the defunct, circa-1980s "Presidential Fitness Patch" awarded to school children for zippy shuttle runs. Make it a coveted digital fitness badge, sans the flexed arm hangs and sit and reach of the prior fitness regimes. Pandemic leadership might have realized a similar effect to the coveted morale-boosting blue arm patches given only to line infantry soldiers during World War II.

Most people are familiar with digital badging, perhaps having earned them for conquering a level in a virtual reality zombie fighting game or earning a work credential such as the free Google Cloud skill badges for learning to code or to manage a serverless platform.[164] Badges work to hack learner motivation.

It was possible.

Just imagine participants encouraged to share their badges and rewards on social media sites, while a timeline and leaderboard displayed on their login page. They could have formed or joined teams. It would have been all the buzz.

The badge progression would have charged participants to develop the knowledge and skills to take responsibility for their own personal fitness and celebrate their accomplishments. This approach also resonates with a point learned when we examined the Iron Soldier earlier. As previously noted, there is doing the right thing, and then there is being seen doing the right thing. It was all there for the taking.

Corporate America might have had a nonpartisan easement to the "we are all in this together" choir by pitching in discount codes for their products or services for people who unlocked special incentives through progress toward their fitness objectives.

Congratulations! This is the tenth day that you logged into your fitness portal. You earned a Tenacity Badge and unlocked a 15% discount code on your next Amazon order. Click to share your badge on your social media platforms!

People would have logged into the Army's Civilian Fitness Program portal, synched their apps and wearable monitors, and reinforced their immune system. Incentives! Goal setting! Self Advocacy! The *Fitness and Fortitude Campaign!*

But there was no such campaign and no such galvanization of the general public toward fitness goals. However, there was plenty of dancing.

HEALTHCARE HEROES AND THE
TIKTOK DANCE CRAZE

In April 2020, at the height of the early pandemic, with 2,000 Americans dying daily, a nurse in America might quickly wrap up his rounds on the intensive care ward or the nursing home—and then join his colleagues in the lobby, hallway, or courtyard where they would spend their lunch breaks in elaborately choreographed dance and song that was recorded and uploaded to social media.

Call it the TikTok Dance Craze of 2020.

In 2018, Will Wilkinson, the writer and intellectual, offered on Twitter that "The cult of 'first responders' is a symptom of a decadent polarized culture groping desperately for somebody we can all agree to esteem."[165] Those words rang even truer during a global pandemic that sorted and slotted us in terms of our usefulness.

There was *essential*, which could mean anything from a truck driver to a clerk at McDonald's to a Shipt shopper, picking up groceries and dropping them off. The *essential* were the people who left home so you did not have to do so.

Then there was the first responder, which is police, the fire department, and medics. First responders are the ones who come fast, with lights and sirens on, when you call 9-1-1. And then, at the top of the pandemic hierarchy, there were nurses.

The first responder has a brief, adrenalized encounter with a person in trauma. A person is picked up from one place, transported to a hospital or a jail or a mental health intake center, and for the first responder, it ends there. But a nurse is in it for the long haul, for however long a hospitalization or convalescence may last.

During a respiratory illness pandemic that required social distancing, and long before the existence of a vaccine, families were locked out of hospitals and nursing homes. This situation meant a nurse might be the last person with whom your aged parent or grandparent had regular in-person contact.

The nurse was not just on the front lines, they were embedded behind them. They were on the same side of the screen door as grandma, as you waved and blew kisses from the other side—from the outside, looking in. With their sickest and most vulnerable loved ones hospitalized and beyond their reach, America gave its nurses a pass when they decided to drown their sorrows in TikTok videos.

If families had any reservations, those were not voiced in the media, which praised the dance routines as morale boosters for people who needed one. *Good Morning America* spoke glowingly of nurse Kala Baker, who "[brought] joy to many by dancing on TikTok."[166]

Nurse.org, a promotion website for the nursing profession, portrayed the dancing as all but necessary. "The strength of nurses in the face of adversity is on clear display in these videos where nurses are shown celebrating the big wins and handling stress in their fight against COVID-19," read one story on five TikTok dance videos that had gone viral.[167]

The dance routines were not the apposite reaction of people at finite voltage. Dance routines were going viral just weeks into the pandemic, long before ninety days was reached. And they were a bit like taking a victory lap while the race was being run.

Before the pandemic, World War II was the last great war America all fought together. The difference between the two shows that the velocity of affirmation is moving at an unprecedented pace. People do not wait until enemies are vanquished anymore to celebrate. They want a down payment on their pain. They want their flowers while they can still smell them.

To drive around in the summer of 1942, with rolling blackouts in American cities employed to get in the practice of denying the enemy lighted targets at night, it would look and feel as though America was at war, even compared to the tough times of the Great Depression.

In the 1930s, someone might have kept the lights off at night to keep their bills low. In 1942, keeping the lights off was a patriotic duty. During a May 1942 partial blackout in Detroit, one apartment building was found to have its lights on throughout, but was discovered to be a company that made calculators. That was "war work," and thus exempt. But otherwise, across several neighborhoods of the city, there was "100% participation" and "not a light showing," *The Detroit News* reported.[168]

In 1946, with flags flying high and veterans walking tall at parades and meat barbecuing and the fat of the land being enjoyed, rather than rationed, one would have seen and felt that the worst was over. Wartime and winning were different, and felt different.

At the start of a pandemic that would kill nearly one million Americans, with death tolls high and victory far from certain, what was there to celebrate? The person staying safe and staying home, scrolling their phone, could rightfully wonder which of the two was true: the news reports of overrun hospitals? Or the all-singing, all-dancing nurses of TikTok?

Were we celebrating, or were we in a pandemic? How could we possibly do both? You could not open the doors of your business due to fears that hospitals would be overrun. But if the hospitals were overrun, how could nurses on the front lines have the time for video shoots?

What was wrong with this picture? And who was watching out for hospitalized grandma during these dance parties? The oversight normally provided by visiting family members was a nonfactor. There was no one to watch the caretakers, and left to their own devices, they shot dance videos.

When the nurses were not celebrating themselves, they were being feted by everyone else—even by the first responders, as Healthcare Heroes parades greeted health workers en route to hospitals, often with police cars, ambulances, and fire trucks announcing their arrival.

In Detroit, ninety first responders from area police and fire agencies formed a caravan parade outside Detroit Receiving Hospital, one of Michigan's busiest emergency hospitals, a place where police are taken when shot in the line of duty. Hospital staff stood outside the entrance to the emergency room and watched.

"Our department was heavily-hit with this COVID disaster," said Commander Darin Szilagy of the Detroit Police Department in an interview with *The Detroit Free Press*. "We can't thank enough our hospital staff and our ERs and our doctors, our nurses, that were really on the front lines and helped us get through."[169]

The Detroit Police Department would have more than 500 of its roughly 2,200 sworn officers quarantined or out sick at some point during the pandemic, including the then-police chief James Craig.[170] And yet it was the first responders who threw the parade for the nurses.

Contrast that scene to the *Road to Victory*: on the *Road to Victory*, it was important everyone saw themselves as playing some role. From the farmer to the stock trader to the warrior.

By contrast, during the pandemic, it was important that all of those people praise nurses. At a solemn time, never was it suggested by a professional board or advocacy group or a thought leader that nurses should tone down the dancing—lest anyone get the wrong idea how serious the pandemic was.

Ironically, of all the nurses in all the TikTok videos during the pandemic, it was one who spoke out, rather than danced, who was punished. Her sin: giving people the wrong idea how serious the pandemic was.

Ashley Grames of Oregon, an oncology nurse, made a November 2020 video with a caption that read: "When my coworkers find out I still travel, don't wear a mask when I am out and let my kids have playdates."[171]

What followed was a firestorm of controversy that caused Grames's employer, Salem Health, to distance itself immediately. She was placed on leave.[172] In the end, going viral the wrong way cost Grames her job, her good name, and, briefly, her profession.

A month after her video, Grames was "prohibited from practicing as a nurse until further notice by the state's nursing board."[173] With a target of public scorn punished publicly, the world moved on from the story. But in March 2021, Grames's license was quietly renewed. There are no disciplinary actions on her file according to the Oregon State Board of Nursing.[174]

Outrage after a viral video has the most finite voltage of all.

DISRUPTING FINITE VOLTAGE: TWELVE WAYS TO BECOME RESILIENT DURING UNCERTAIN TIMES

We can do things to strengthen ourselves, for each of us to become more resilient to finite voltage.

Individual resilience is important to community resilience in that healthy people make for a healthier community. Healthy communities are better able to manage and recover from disasters and other emergencies.[175]

Here are twelve ways to strengthen resilience during uncertain times.

1. **"I observed"**

   When describing something, communicate your personal observations of what you saw, heard, or felt. Saying, "I observed" is empowering and typically more accurate than repeating second-hand information. You will practice "I observed" framing as part of a member check network.

2. **Embrace crowd-in**

   Humans are hard-wired to worry. But if the problem cannot be solved, languishing in the worry-world will be exhausting. It is acceptable to surround yourself with things that make you feel comfortable during uncertain times. We will learn more about crowd-in behavior in part 5.

3. **Name your fears or experiences (paradoxical intention)**

   Remember the torus and how humans will do almost anything to ensure that things stay the same? We are scared of the unknown. By naming things, like "finite voltage" or applying Clay Martin's "Cracked Board experience," vague fears and unspoken taboos lose their ability to control you.

4. **Identify and mitigate sources of "noise"**

   In the Linda Stone chapter, we learned the importance of attention hygiene. Excess or constant audio, visual, or psychological stimuli burdens our attention and leads to cognitive fatigue. Turn off the TV, silence your phone, and cleanse your mind with a stroll in the park.

5. **Talk to yourself in the third person (Socratic dialogue)**

   Research suggests that talking to yourself in the third person can be an effective form of self-control.[176] The next time you need to make a decision during an emotional moment, take a moment to talk silently to yourself using the third person. It might help you stay calm, collected, and level-headed, a strategy that may prevent bad decisions made in the heat of the moment.

6. **Parkinson's Law—Restore start and end routines**

   Having a routine is helpful during uncertain times because it gives you a sense of control over the events of your life. Routines and schedules also provide a transitory benefit as we complete tasks and activities with satisfaction and then move forward to other things; new things are often accompanied by a sense of optimism and energy.

7. **Change things every sixty days**

   The "sameness" of each day, combined with a loss of routine and fewer opportunities for novel experiences like going on a trip or eating at a restaurant, makes most people perceive time as passing slowly. In these instances, setting goals at sixty-day intervals will quell the listless drift, create unique experiences, and give you direction. Here are three campaigns to power you through half of a year: Get fit, read books, learn to cook!

8. **Expressive writing or creations of art (or something)**

   Writing organizes our thoughts and helps us cope with situations. It might be a diary, letter, observations, a story, or whatever is on your mind. By dating journal entries, we demonstrate transition forward through time. Likewise, art encourages creative thinking, a sense of control, and a feeling of accomplishment. Making art can also be a comforting crowd-in behavior.

9. **Images over words**

   As we examined in the Committee for National Morale's *Road to Victory* campaign, communicating visually can simplify messaging when people are overwhelmed by stressful situations. "Pictures are not only more effortless to recognize and process than words, but also easier to recall. When words enter long-term memory they do so with a single code. Pictures, on the other hand, contain two codes: one visual and the other verbal, each stored in different places in the brain."[177]

10. **Social network**

In his book *Happiness: Lessons from a New Science*, economist Richard Layard indicated that if one excludes personality and genes as explanatory factors, social relations are among the most important determinants of well-being.[178] "People who enjoy close relationships are found to cope better with various types of stress, including job loss and illness."[179]

11. **Exercise, nutrition, and sleep**

The law of entropy means that the natural tendency of systems is to become increasingly disordered over time. When prolonged, unsettled circumstances disrupt exercise, nutrition, and sleep, our bodies are weakened and vulnerable to physical and cognitive entropy. Fortunately, we learned in the Home Front Morale in 2020—Fitness and Fortitude segment that tending to our fitness alleviates stress and strengthens our immune systems. Fitness is inclusive, regardless of proficiency. According to professional strength trainer Drew Baye, "If you can contract your muscles voluntarily, you can exercise."[180]

12. **Spend more time outdoors**

"Research has shown that spending time in nature has been associated with decreased levels of mental illness, with the strongest links to reduced symptoms of depression and anxiety, in addition to increased self-esteem."[181] In the general population, other studies have shown that *attention* is almost uniformly enhanced by exposure to natural environments. University of Michigan psychology researchers Marc Berman, John Jonides, and Stephen Kaplan found memory performance and attention spans improved by 20 percent after people spent an hour interacting with nature.[182]

There is much we can do to preserve our personal well-being weeks or months into a stressful situation. It is rare for chaos conditions to last more than ninety days. When they do, there is often a population-level "sense" that the event might not be transitory in nature. In other words, we are not able to predict when it might end, or are not confident that our lives will be similar to how they were before this prolonged state of unsettled times.

In chapter 5, we will learn of what happens at a population level when chaos continues beyond three months and how crowd-in behavior signals a change in how people perceive their future.

NOTES

1. Nikolai Razouvaev, personal communications with the author, January 2021 to April 2021.

2. United States Department of Defense. "Joint Fire Support." Joint Publication 3-09. April 10, 2019. https://www.jcs.mil/Portals/36/Documents/Doctrine/pubs/jp3 _09.pdf?ver=2019-05-14-081632-887.

3. Dickson, James. "Suspects Arrested in Warren Shooting Tracked by Cell Phone to Wayne." The Detroit News. April 28, 2020. https://www.detroitnews.com /story/news/local/macomb-county/2020/04/28/suspects-arrested-warren-shooting -tracked-cellphone-wayne/3038347001/.

4. Aaron Sawyer, interview with the author, August 14, 2020.

5. City of Chicago. "Reopening Chicago." City of Chicago. 2020. https://www .chicago.gov/city/en/sites/COVID-19/home/reopening-chicago.html.

6. Sawyer, interview with the author.

7. Parkinson, Cyril Northcote. *Parkinson's Law [And Other Studies in Administration]* (Cambridge, MA: The Riverside Press, 1957), 3. http://sas2.elte.hu/ tg/ptorv/Parkinson-s-Law.pdf.

8. Linda Stone, personal communication with the author, August 14, 2020.

9. Sawyer, interview with the author.

10. Ibid.

11. Ibid.

12. Ibid.

13. Bureau of Labor Statistics. "Supplemental Data Measuring the Effects of the Coronavirus (COVID-19) Pandemic on the Labor Market." Labor Force Statistics from the Current Population Survey. Bureau of Labor Statistics. Last Modified September 10, 2021. https://www.bls.gov/cps/effects-of-the-coronavirus-COVID-19 -pandemic.htm.

14. Sawyer, interview with the author.

15. Ibid.

16. Ibid.

17. Ibid.

18. Ibid.

19. Ibid.

20. Appel, John. *Fighting Fear: The Role of Psychiatrists in World War II* (Rockville, MD: American Heritage, October 1999), 1.

21. Appel, *Fighting Fear*, 1.

22. Ibid.

23. Ibid.

24. Ibid.

25. Appel, *Fighting Fear*, 2.

26. Ibid.

27. Ibid.

28. Ibid.

29. Ibid.

30. Ibid., 1.

31. Ibid., 2. Behringer, Ashley. "Why We Fight: Prelude to War, America's Crash History Lesson." U.S. Archives. September 1, 2020. https://unwritten-record .blogs.archives.gov/2020/09/01/why-we-fight-prelude-to-war-americas-crash-history -lesson/.

32. United States Department of Defense. "Why We Fight: Prelude to War." Directed by Frank Capra. May 27, 1942.

33. Appel, *Fighting Fear*, 5.

34. Ibid., 4.

35. Sobel, Raymond. "The 'Old Sergeant' Syndrome." *Psychiatry* 10, no. 3 (1947): 315. doi: 10.1080/00332747.1947.11022649.

36. Appel, *Fighting Fear*, 5.

37. Ibid.

38. Ibid.

39. Pearl Harbor Warbirds. "Top 18 Vintage WWII Pinup Poster Girls." PearlHarborWarbirds.com. May 7, 2015. https://pearlharborwarbirds.com/vintage-wwii-pinup-poster-girls/.

40. Appel, *Fighting Fear*, 3.

41. Ibid., 4.

42. Ibid.

43. Clay Martin, personal communication with the author, January 23, 2021.

44. Clay Martin, personal communication.

45. Clay Martin, "Clay Martin: Author of Concrete Jungle: A Green Beret's Guide to Urban Survival." Interview by David P. Perrodin. *The Safety Doc Podcast.* July 18, 2020. https://www.youtube.com/watch?v=sv35UvI3JZE.

46. Martin, *Author of Concrete Jungle*.

47. Gray Wolf Survival. "Using Kim's Game to Train Your Mind for Survival." GrayWolfSurvival.com. August 26, 2014. https://graywolfsurvival.com/2173/using-kims-game-to-train-your-mind-for-survival/.

48. Martin, *Author of Concrete Jungle*.

49. U.S. Army. "U.S. Army Prepping Newest Robin Sage Exercise." The Pilot. March 24, 2021. https://www.thepilot.com/news/army-prepping-newest-robin-sage-exercise/article_9125fd6c-8ca1-11eb-a0b6-2f015a9aea2a.html.

50. Martin, *Author of Concrete Jungle*.

51. Ibid.

52. Delaney Williams, "Refugees," The Wire, Season 04, Episode 04, directed by David Simon. Original Air Date October 1, 2006 (Baltimore, MD: HBO, 2006).

53. Clay Martin, personal communication with the author, May 14, 2021.

54. Clay Martin, personal communication.

55. Ibid.

56. Ibid.

57. Ibid.

58. Ibid.

59. Ibid.

60. Martin, *Author of Concrete Jungle*.

61. Ibid.

62. Clay Martin, personal communication with the author, January 23, 2021.

63. Clay Martin, personal communication.

64. Ibid.

65. Ibid.

66. Ibid.

67. Ibid.

68. Ibid.

69. Ibid.

70. Janocha, Jill. "Facts of the Catch: Occupational Injuries, Illnesses, and Fatalities to Fishing Workers, 2003-2009." Beyond the Numbers: Workplace Injuries, vol. 1, no. 9. August 2012. https://www.bls.gov/opub/btn/volume-1/facts-of-the-catch -occupational-injuries-illnesses-and-fatalities-to-fishing-workers-2003-2009.htm.

71. Janocha, *Facts of the Catch.*

72. Martin, personal communication.

73. Ibid.

74. Ibid.

75. Ibid.

76. Ibid.

77. Ibid.

78. Ibid.

79. Ibid.

80. Ibid.

81. Ibid.

82. Ibid.

83. Ibid.

84. Ibid.

85. Ibid.

86. Janocha, *Facts of the Catch.*

87. Martin, personal communication.

88. Ibid.

89. Krugel, Lauren. "Fort McMurray Wildfire Named Canada's News Story of 2016." The Canadian Press. December 20, 2016. https://globalnews.ca/news/3138183 /fort-mcmurray-wildfire-named-canadas-news-story-of-2016/.

90. Goss, Hilton. *Civilian Morale During Aerial Bombardment, 1917-1939* (Maxwell Air Force Base, Montgomery, AL: Air University, 1948), 5.

91. Black, Annetta. "Wehrmann in Eisen Nail Man." Atlas Obscura. January 13, 2013. https://www.atlasobscura.com/places/wehrmann-in-eisen-nail-man.

92. Black, *Wehrmann in Eisen.*

93. Cornwall, Mark. "Propaganda at Home, Austria-Hungary." International Encyclopedia of the First World War. April 25, 2019.

94. Committee on Public Information. "The Four-Minute Men. Bulleting No. 1." Committee on Public Information. May 22, 1917. https://catalog.hathitrust.org/ Record/006785210.

95. Ibid.

96. National Center for Education Statistics (NCES). "120 Years of Literacy. Illiteracy." September 1992. https://nces.ed.gov/naal/lit_history.asp#illiteracy.

97. The Topeka Daily Capital. "Four-Minute Men to Stir Patriotic Blood of Kansas." The Topeka Daily Capital. September 1, 1917.

98. The Topeka Daily Capital, *Four-Minute Men.*

99. Ibid.

100. Monger, David. "Propaganda at Home (Great Britain and Ireland, Version)." International Encyclopedia of the First World War. Last Updated January 8, 2017, 2. https://encyclopedia.1914-1918-online.net/article/propaganda_at_home_great_britain_and_ireland.

101. Cummans, Jared. "A Brief History of Bond Investing." BondFunds.com. October 1, 2014. http://bondfunds.com/education/a-brief-history-of-bond-investing/.

102. Castagnetti, Sarah. "Every Little Helps: The History of the National Savings Movement." The U.K. National Archives. May 11, 2020. https://blog.nationalarchives.gov.uk/every-little-helps-the-history-of-the-national-savings-movement/.

103. Ryfe, David Michael. "From Media Audience to Media Public: A Study of Letters Written in Reaction to FDR's Fireside Chats." *Media, Culture and Society* 23 (November 1, 2001): 767–781. doi: 10.1177/016344301023006005.

104. History.com Editors. "FDR Broadcasts First 'Fireside Chat' During the Great Depression." History.com. November 24, 2009. https://www.history.com/this-day-in-history/fdr-gives-first-fireside-chat.

105. Ryfe, *From Media Audience to Media Public*, 767–781.

106. Ibid.

107. Snyder, Louis L. and Richard B. Morris. *A Treasury of Great Reporting: "Literature Under Pressure" From the 16th Century to Our Own Time* (New York: Simon and Shuster, 1949), 126–128.

108. Lim, Elvin T. "The Lion and the Lamb: Demythologizing Franklin Roosevelt's Fireside Chats." *Rhetoric and Public Affairs* 6, no. 3 (February, 2003): 438–464.

109. Lim, *The Lion and the Lamb,* 438–464.

110. Slotkin, Jason. "Biden Revives Weekly Presidential Tradition, Releasing First Weekly Address." NPR. February 6, 2021. https://www.npr.org/2021/02/06/964889898/biden-revives-presidential-tradition-releasing-first-weekly-address.

111. Lim, *The Lion and the Lamb*, 438–464.

112. APM Reports. "Letters to Franklin Delano Roosevelt." APMReports.org. November 10, 2014. https://www.apmreports.org/episode/2014/11/10/letters-to-franklin-delano-roosevelt.

113. APM Reports. "Letters to Franklin Delano Roosevelt, Melvin J. Chisum, October 1, 1934." APM Reports. November 10, 2014. https://www.apmreports.org/episode/2014/11/10/letters-to-franklin-delano-roosevelt.

114. APM Reports. "Letters to Franklin Delano Roosevelt, Hugh F. Colliton, Jr., October 1, 1934." APM Reports. November 10, 2014. https://www.apmreports.org/episode/2014/11/10/letters-to-franklin-delano-roosevelt.

115. Sandburg, Carl. "Road to Victory, A Procession of Photographs of the Nation at War." Directed by Lt. Comdr. Edward Steichen, U.S.N.R. Museum of Modern Art, New York, 1942, 12.

116. Sterling, Christopher H. "The Fireside Chats: President Franklin D. Roosevelt, 1933-1944." The Library of Congress. 2002. https://www.loc.gov/static/programs/national-recording-preservation-board/documents/FiresideChats.pdf.

117. Herman, Ellen. *The Romance of American Psychology: Political Culture in the Age of Experts* (Berkeley: University of California Press, 1995), 49.

118. Herman, *The Romance of American Psychology,* 49.

119. Newmeyer, Sarah. "Press Release: Two Famous Americans Arrange Road to Victory Exhibition at Museum of Modern Art." Museum of Modern Art. May 13, 1942. https://www.moma.org/momaorg/shared/pdfs/docs/press_archives/796/releases/MOMA_1942_0038_1942-05-13_42513-32.pdf.

120. Fred Turner, "Your Undivided Attention 23: When Media Was For You and Me." Interviewed by Tristan Harris. *The Undivided Attention Podcast.* August 5, 2020. https://www.humanetech.com/podcast/23-when-media-was-for-you-and-me.

121. Fred Turner, *When Media Was For You and Me.*

122. Ibid.

123. Ibid.

124. Ibid.

125. Ibid.

126. Ibid.

127. Sandburg, *Road to Victory.*

128. Neumeyer, Sarah, *Press Release: Two Famous Americans.*

129. Sandburg, *Road to Victory.*

130. Ibid.

131. Fred Turner, *When Media Was For You and Me.*

132. Ibid.

133. @SafetyPhD. "Bellevue, WA has an ONLINE TOOL to report Social Distancing Violation!" Twitter. March, 31, 2020. https://twitter.com/SafetyPhD/status/1245065591809028096.

134. Dr. David Mays, private interview by David P. Perrodin, May 28, 2021.

135. Dr. David Mays, private interview.

136. Ibid.

137. Ibid.

138. Ibid.

139. Ibid.

140. Ibid.

141. Ibid.

142. Ibid.

143. LeBlanc, Beth, Craig Mauger, and Melissa Nann Burke. "High Court Strikes Down Whitmer's Emergency Powers; Gov Vows to Use Other Means." The Detroit News. October 2, 2020. https://www.detroitnews.com/story/news/local/michigan/2020/10/02/michigan-supreme-court-strikes-down-gretchen-whitmers-emergency-powers/5863340002.

144. Chappell, Bill. "New York Legislature Strips Cuomo of Extraordinary Emergency Powers, With a Caveat." NPR. March 5, 2021. https://www.npr.org/2021/03/05/974083354/new-york-legislature-strips-cuomo-of-extraordinary-emergency-powers-with-a-caveat.

145. Lovelace, Jr., Berkeley. "CDC Says Fully Vaccinated People Don't Need to Wear Face Masks Indoors or Outdoors in Most Settings." CNBC.com. May 13, 2021. https://www.cnbc.com/2021/05/13/cdc-says-fully-vaccinated-people-dont-need-to-wear-face-masks-indoors-or-outdoors-in-most-settings.html.

146. The New York Times. "Coronavirus in the U.S. Latest Map and Case Count." The New York Times. May 13, 2021. https://www.nytimes.com/interactive/2021/us/covid-cases.html.

147. Dr. David Mays, private interview.

148. Ibid.

149. Ibid.

150. Ibid.

151. Center for Health Security. Event 201. Johns Hopkins Bloomberg School of Public Health. 2021. https://www.centerforhealthsecurity.org/event201/.

152. Center for Health Security. Event 201, Players. Johns Hopkins Bloomberg School of Public Health. 2021. https://www.centerforhealthsecurity.org/event201/players/.

153. Taylor, Derrick Bryson. "A Timeline of the Coronavirus Pandemic." The New York Times. March 17, 2021. https://www.nytimes.com/article/coronavirus -timeline.html.

154. The Johns Hopkins Center for Health Security. "Event 201 Pandemic Exercise: Highlights Reel." YouTube. November 9, 2019. https://youtu.be/AoLw -Q8X174.

155. Center for Health Security. Event 201, Resources. Johns Hopkins Bloomberg School of Public Health. 2021. https://www.centerforhealthsecurity.org/event201/resources/.

156. Center for Health Security. Event 201, Recommendations. Johns Hopkins Bloomberg School of Public Health. 2021. https://www.centerforhealthsecurity.org/event201/recommendations.html.

157. Center for Health Security, *Event 201 Recommendations*.

158. Brueck, Hilary. "Forget Vitamins: Fauci Says the 3 Best Things 'To Keep Your Immune System Working Optimally' Cost Nothing." Business Insider. September 17, 2020. https://www.businessinsider.com/fauci-3-tips-keep-your -immune-system-strong-vitamins-sleep-2020-9.

159. da Silveira, Matheus Pelinski, Kimberly Kamila da Silva Fagundes, Matheus Ribeiro Bizuti, Édina Starck, Renata Calciolari Rossi, and Débora Tavares de Resende e Silva. "Physical Exercise as a Tool to Help the Immune System Against COVID-19: An Integrative Review of the Current Literature." *Clinical and Experimental Medicine* 1, no. 14 (July 29, 2020): 1. doi: 10.1007/s10238-020-00650-3.

160. Novobilski, Marisa. "Get Moving, Get Fit with Army Civilian Fitness Program." U.S. Army. May 1, 2015. https://www.army.mil/article/147690/get_moving_get_fit_with_army_civilian_fitness_program.

161. Novobilski, *Get Moving, Get Fit*.

162. Drew Baye, "Strength Trainer Drew Baye: Is Student Fitness Sapping School Safety?" Interview by David P. Perrodin. *The Safety Doc Podcast*. February 28, 2020. http://safetyphd.com/safety-doc-podcast-119-strength-trainer-drew-baye-is-student -fitness-sapping-school-safety-podcast/.

163. Drew Baye, *Strength Trainer Drew Baye*.

164. Hartzell, Taryn. "Learn to Code for the Cloud: Earn Native App Development Skills Badges for Free." Google.com. July 8, 2021. https://cloud.google.com/

blog/topics/training-certifications/introducing-new-native-app-development-skills
-challenge.

165. Wilkinson, Will. "The Cult of 'First Responders' is a Symptom of a Decadent Polarized Culture Groping Desperately for *Somebody* We Can All Agree to Esteem." @WillWilkinson, Twitter.com. https://twitter.com/willwilkinson/status /960327206407954432.

166. Good Morning America. "Nurse Kala Baker Brings Joy to Many by Dancing on TikTok." ABC News. April 1, 2020. https://abcnews.go.com/GMA/Wellness/ video/nurse-kala-baker-brings-joy-dancing-tiktok-69912394.

167. Jividen, Sarah. "5 Videos of Dancing Nurses Go Viral in Celebration of Recovered COVID-19 Patients." Nurse.org. April 23, 2020. https://nurse.org/articles /nurses-viral-tiktok-social-media-covid19-videos/.

168. The Detroit News. "Sunday's Darkening Praised." The Detroit News. May 4, 1942.

169. Detroit Free Press. "Detroit-Area Law Enforcement Form a Parade to Honor Healthcare Heroes." YouTube. April 18, 2020. https://www.youtube.com/watch?v =g674KOSRlsg.

170. Fox 2 Detroit. "Almost 500 Detroit Police Officers Quarantined for Possible Coronavirus. Coronavirus in Michigan." Fox 2 Detroit. March 30, 2020. https:// www.fox2detroit.com/news/almost-500-detroit-police-officers-quarantined-for-pos-sible-coronavirus. Elrick, M. L., Tresa Baldas, and Gina Kaufman. "152 Detroit Police Quarantined Amid Coronavirus Outbreak, 5 Test Positive." Detroit Free Press. March 20, 2020. https://www.freep.com/story/news/local/michigan/detroit/2020/03 /20/detroit-police-coronavirus/2884695001/.

171. Toropin, Konstantin, Allen Kim, and Leah Asmelash. "Nurse Who Bragged About Breaking COVID-19 Rules on TikTok Has Lost Her Job." CNNWire. CNN. December 8, 2020. https://abc7news.com/8613919/.

172. Marine, Drew. "Salem Health Addresses Controversial TikTok Posted by Nurse." KPTV-TV. November 29, 2020. https://www.kptv.com/news/salem-health -addresses-controversial-tiktok-posted-by-nurse/article_8fcda1a0-321e-11eb-ac91 -5bbd017ce2a9.html.

173. Nashrulla, Tasneem. "The Oregon Nurse Who Bragged on TikTok About Breaking COVID-19 Restrictions Has Agreed to Stop Practicing." Buzzfeed. December 7, 2020. https://www.buzzfeednews.com/article/tasneemnashrulla/oregon -nurse-covid-tiktok-salem-hospital.

174. Oregon State Board of Nursing. "Verification of Licensure for Ashley Grames." Oregon State Board of Nursing. May 10, 2021. https://osbn.oregon.gov/ osbnverification/Details.aspx?person=79626c9e-77dd-df11-af93-0021f6000008.

175. United States Department of Health and Human Services. "Individual Resilience." Public Health Emergency: Public Health and Medical Emergency Support for a Nation Prepared. United States Department of Health and Human Services. Last Reviewed September 8, 2020. https://www.phe.gov/Preparedness/ planning/abc/Pages/individual-resilience.aspx.

176. Moser, Jason S., Adrienne Dougherty, Whitney I. Mattson, Benjamin Katz, Tim P. Moran, Darwin Guevarra, Holly Shablack, Ozlem Ayduk, John Jonides, Marc G. Berman, and Ethan Kross. "Third Person Self-Talk Facilitates Emotion Regulation

Without Engaging Cognitive Control: Converging Evidence from ERP and fMRI." *Scientific Reports* 7, no. 1(4519) (July 3, 2017): doi: 10.1038/s41598-017-04047-3.

177. Dewan, Pauline. "Words Versus Pictures: Leveraging the Research on Visual Communication." *The Canadian Journal of Library and Information Practices and Research* 10, no. 1 (June 15, 2015): 2.

178. Layard, Richard, *Happiness: Lessons From a New Science* (London: Penguin Books, 2005).

179. van der Horst, Mariska, and Hilde Coffe. "How Friendship Network Characteristics Influence Subjective Well-Being." *Social Indicators Research* 107, no. 3 (July 2012): 512. doi: 10.1007%2Fs11205-011-9861-2.

180. Drew Baye, *Strength Trainer Drew Baye.*

181. Preston, Susanne. "Spending Time in Nature for Your Health—How Outdoor Activities Improve Wellbeing." Counseling and Psychology. South University. August 23, 2016. https://www.southuniversity.edu/news-and-blogs/2016/08/spending-time-in-nature-for-your-health-how-outdoor-activities-improve-wellbeing-102984.

182. Berman, Marc, John Jonides, and Stephen Kaplan. "Going Outside—Even in the Cold—Improves Memory, Attention." University of Michigan. December 16, 2008. https://news.umich.edu/going-outsideeven-in-the-coldimproves-memory-attention/.

Chapter 5

Crowd-In Behavior

In 1981, Faith Popcorn, recognized as America's foremost trend expert, coined the term *Cocooning*.[1] (*Cocooning* is analogous to the term *crowd-in behavior* used in this book.)

Popcorn defined *cocooning* as "The need to protect oneself from the harsh, unpredictable realities of the outside world."[2] It described how we looked for psychological shelter, and it continues to. But what began as something cozy has become self-preservation in this age of pandemics.[3]

HYGEE: THE DANISH MINDSET

Christmas decor cocooned people in a colorful, cozy slice of joy insulated from the misery of the pandemic, civil unrest, and economic woes that fell outside and the long, dark, chilled winter months that routinely sank people's moods.

We heard people justify their pause to shift the holiday gears, noting that holiday decorations defused positive energy or keeping them in sight was some type of "mental health strategy."

According to the American Academy of Family Physicians, approximately 4 to 6 percent of people may have winter depression.[4] Another 10 to 20 percent may have mild seasonal affective disorder (SAD).[5] Some symptoms of SAD include: decreased energy, fatigue, problems sleeping, having difficulty concentrating, social withdrawal, and feeling hopeless or worthless.

The Mayo Clinic's recommendations for treating SAD include making your environment sunnier and brighter and getting outside.[6] And what is brighter than a tree adorned with a 1,000 lights? Maybe bringing the outside inside and lighting it up and keeping it up is something we should have made socially acceptable years ago—at least outside Scandinavia.

With up to seventeen hours of darkness and long, cold winters, Denmark's harsh weather does not chill the happiness of its citizens. According to the 2021 *World Happiness Report* which ranks countries by how happy their citizens perceive themselves, Denmark was ranked second, behind Finland.[7]

Danes have practiced the concept of *hygge* for hundreds of years. Perhaps at one time it was a coping mechanism to countervail the trickster antics of mythical Norse chaos god Loki.

Hygge is a concept originated in Danish culture that focuses on living with a sense of comfort, coziness, and peace. It has been described as, "creating a warm atmosphere and enjoying the good things in life with good people."[8]

Lore has it that hygge boosted Danes through abysmal winters as they chose to surround themselves with comfort items such as candles, wooly socks, decorations, and bright colors.

Hygge differs from chaos-driven crowd-in behavior in a few ways. First, hygge is not preceded by a finite voltage event. Inasmuch as Scandinavian winters are feats of endurance, they are predictable and yield to spring by the end of March. Second, hygge is not a winter-only phenomenon. It is practiced year-round. And third, crowd-in behavior involves surrounding oneself with comfort items, but the general feeling is of worry and uncertainty for the future. People embracing hygge, on the other hand, are relaxed and think positively, both about the present and toward the future.

Helen Russell, author of *The Year of Living Danishly: Uncovering the Secrets of the World's Happiest Country*, stated, "My most hygge experience to date was probably watching the sun set from a hot tub in a blizzard in January, beer in hand."[9]

Western culture retailers, with sales calendars in lockstep to holidays and seasons, have recently embraced the fairly wide open commerce opportunities of a hygge mindset.

Just in time, the algorithms replaced advertisements for twinkling Christmas lights with twinkling lighted "(faux) birch trees," available in sizes from 12 inches to 8 feet! And people quickly purchased them; right along with the assorted "ornaments" also available for Valentine's Day, St. Patrick's Day, and even Easter. No one questioned having this new type of tree indoors. There was simply joy that whatever reprieve the holidays had brought, that joyous feeling (like the pandemic) was not over yet.

The practice of hygee is a perennial approach to managing negative long-term impacts. But what happens when we confuse short-term solutions with long-term impacts from crowding-in behavior?

POOCHES, PILLOWS, POOLS, AND PUZZLES

Under orders to stay home and stay safe, in a time of pandemic, isolated people found the affection they craved for at the pet store. Forced to be socially distant from what would normally bring them comfort—friends, family, church, restaurants, travel, gym—people adopted furry friends in massive numbers in 2020. So great was the demand for pets that some animal shelters ran out, reported *The Washington Post.*[10]

And why not? If you were going to be home for a while, with duration to-be-determined, why not fill that home with love? And what about your house? That inner-ring starter home that made sense when your kid was a baby, when half your waking hours were spent elsewhere, and before the dog. Now, it is a tight fit.

You never anticipated that home would someday double as your workplace, your gym, and a one-room schoolhouse for your kids. If the house you call home must serve multiple purposes, why not get a space big enough to do so? National Public Radio (NPR) reported in August 2020 that "despite the steepest plunge into a recession on record, historically high unemployment and an uncertain outlook for the economy, the housing market is on a tear."[11]

If you did not have a pool in your backyard before the pandemic, you probably did not think you needed one. You did not need the cost, the maintenance, the company, or the potential liability. If ever you needed waterfront rest and relaxation, you would travel to poolside Vegas or the beach.

As far as you were concerned, all the life worth living was out in the world, beyond your property line. But when you are staring at a summer without travel, and possibly two summers, a dip in your own pool on a hot day does not sound half-bad.

And as *The New York Times* found, crowd-in behaviors do not just take place in isolation.[12] Envy can play a role, too. At work, people come to the same place. On Zoom, working from home, the differing quality of those homes jumps off the screen.

Reenat Sinay, a journalist in Manhattan, told *The New York Times* she had grown covetous from her electronic windows into how people live elsewhere, with more space and cheaper rent.[13] "There is one woman on my team who is engaged and has this gorgeous apartment with this awesome balcony," Sinay told *The New York Times*. "She always Zooms from there and I'm always like, 'Damn.'"[14]

The dog, the house in the outer-ring suburbs, and the in-ground pool are three physical manifestations of crowd-in behavior. We crowd-in when we are seeking comfort in a season of unpleasantness.

In March 2020, the world changed overnight. Suddenly, our access to work, to church, and to visit family members was decided by state governors or shared at press conferences, with few questions and no debate. We were told that the very act of leaving home risked the spread of a deadly global virus.

If change is hard, overnight change is that much more difficult. The mind tries every trick it can to deny that things have changed. After denial, comes acceptance, and after acceptance comes crowd-in behavior. It is the sugar that makes the medicine go down.

Crowd-in behaviors are primarily exhibited by rule-followers who are steeling themselves for a hard journey they have accepted but did not choose. The dog, the house, and the pool matter more to someone who will be staying home as ordered than to someone who never stops traveling.

Scofflaws do not crowd-in; nothing has changed for them. Crowd-in behavior is a coping mechanism.

To be sure, there were also less-permanent versions of crowding-in during the pandemic, including Netflix and chill, baking sourdough bread, and the purchase and completion of elaborate puzzles.[15] NPR reported that jigsaw sales were up 300 percent at points in the early pandemic.[16]

Chris Byrne, "The Toy Guy," explained to NPR why puzzles found a rebirth amid crisis:

> It really takes your focus off of whatever's going on, because you're trying to find that peak of the barn or that piece of sky or this element of cloud. . . . It really takes a lot of attention and focus. And that can be very healthy in terms of, I'll just say, distraction.[17]

But it is at the extreme end that the coping nature of crowd-in behavior is most obvious. People make permanent decisions to cope with temporary circumstances. The dogs will live longer than the pandemic will last. A fifteen- or thirty-year mortgage will far outlast the space crunch that necessitated it. And that pool could have been a year of law school for your kid.

So great is the human need to cope that crowd-in behaviors can be life-affecting decisions.

"Dad, Can I Borrow the Webcam?"

Business Insider reported webcams among ten unlikely items that sold well during the pandemic.[18] Some people needed them for work as meetings that were face-to-face moved online. Others, with time away from work, found the need to express themselves to the world.

With a webcam, you could reach grandma, the office, clients, or family and friends a world away. There was also good business to be done. In March 2020, two rap producers named Timbaland and Swizz Beatz faced off in a battle called Verzuz.[19] On Instagram, the two would perform or songs, and the crowd would decide who won.

As described in *New York Magazine*, "Verzuz reimagines the of hip-hop's early days for the 'one gotta go' set."[20] Verzuz was crowd-in behavior taken global. Urging people to stay home and stay safe is one thing. Giving people appointment programming that would keep them home is quite another.

More than a year later, Verzuz is a full-blown brand. Such is the power of crowding-in around a webcam.

Panic-Buying and Survivalism

Crowd-in behavior must be distinguished from what it is not: panic-buying. People panic-buy paper towels and bleach wipes for everything from pandemics to bad weather reports. However, people do not buy dogs for companionship after a hurricane hits, as conditions are not secure enough to bring another life into the mix. Panic-buying is loading up on canned pasta at the grocery store because you are not sure where your next meal will come from, when you will have power, or when life will return to normal.

Crowd-in behavior is installing a wood-fired oven because you know you will be cooking your own pizza for a while. Nor can crowd-in behavior be confused with a run on ammo, or guns, or even people joining survivalist militias. These behaviors are better classified as doomsday prep.

People crowding-in do not believe they are in a doomsday scenario. They know life has changed, and not for the better, but have found a means to exert control within their New Normal. The dog, the house, and the pool all mean it cannot be doomsday quite yet. There are too many bills still to pay.

As a Cambridge, Massachusetts woman told *The New York Times*, after upgrading old furniture that was thought tolerable once upon a time, but became an obvious eyesore during the pandemic: "If I'm going to be here, I want it to be as comfortable as possible and as calming as possible."[21]

Distinguishing crowding-in behavior from survivalism becomes even more critical when additional chaos events compound an existing chaos event.

AUTONOMOUS ZONES, MORGAN ROGUE, AND VINDICATION OF THE PREPPER

So now you have the dog, the house, and the in-ground pool of your dreams. If you are going to be home, it might as well be the house you want, with the accommodations you want. Got it. But COVID-19 wasn't the only shock to our sense of safety in 2020. In the wake of George Floyd's Memorial Day death, during his arrest by Minneapolis police, protesters across America took to the street for months.

After Floyd's death, in Detroit, which was still (incredibly) rebuilding from the 1967 riot, protests lasted months, but were largely peaceful. By contrast, in 2020, downtown Minneapolis burned, including an entire police precinct torched to the ground. Portland's federal courthouse burned multiple times. A section of Seattle was briefly claimed by rioters as the Capitol Hill Autonomous Zone, or CHAZ.

Television cameras and smartphone live-streams caught it all, including a New Normal formed before our eyes in Seattle. CHAZ was not just tacitly allowed to operate, wink-wink. It was openly condoned by Mayor Jenny Durkan, who portrayed the siege of a section of her city as a "block party atmosphere," one that "could turn into a summer of love," if the adults did not meddle too much.[22] "It's not an armed takeover," Durkan told CNN's Chris Cuomo. "It's not a military junta."[23]

A Seattle police station was within the autonomous zone, and the city briefly allowed its annexation. Asked how long the autonomous zone might last, Durkan said: "I don't know. We could have the Summer of Love." Then, reality set in. After the autonomous zone, now renamed CHOP—the Capitol Hill Organized Protest area—started racking up a crime rate, Seattle police broke it up.

"What has happened here on these streets over the last two weeks—few weeks, that is—is lawless, and it's brutal, and bottom line, it is simply unacceptable," said Seattle Police Chief Carmen Best, as officers retook the area.[24] The Summer of Love zeitgeist was over. By December, so was Durkan's political career when she announced she would not run for re-election.[25]

You Say You Want a Revolution

Injustice-related unrest is nothing new in America, but in 2020 it took on a different flavor. This time, it fanned out beyond city hall, beyond downtown business districts. This time, protesters marched directly into residential neighborhoods and suburbs, and even into gated communities designed specifically to keep outsiders away.[26]

The revolution was not just televised or tweeted out—do not look now; it is walking down your street, chanting, and demanding that you chant. Neighborhood-based protests were *meant* to be invasive.

They had that effect, and for many people it was a wake-up call that the dog, the home, and the in-ground pool were under greater threat than they had imagined when buying that house in a tree-lined suburb. Not even the outer-ring suburbs were exempt. No one could be assured that the revolution would not come to their doorstep.

What if your home was in that autonomous zone? Or your business? What if the ground under your feet was annexed and assigned to angry people by politicians reading tea leaves? What if you needed help and the police and EMS would not even make 9-1-1 runs to where you were?

While protesters in Seattle declared their autonomy from the city, homesteaders, preppers, and homeschoolers across America worked to be independent of a food system, a social order, and an education system in which they had lost faith. High food prices and empty shelves became indicators of a possible food scarcity.

For many people, planning for the future meant *canning* for the future—so much so that mason jars were in short supply at points during the pandemic.[27] This supply shortage was not the stuff of selfies, like the sourdough. People prepare canned food because they will actually need that food at some future point.

Going Rogue

Morgan Rogue, survivalist extraordinaire, was prepping before it was cool. The owner of Rogue Preparedness, Rogue shepherds people through their survivalist journey.[28] Her motto: "conquer tomorrow by preparing today."[29] The Rogue Preparedness YouTube channel has amassed 31,000 subscribers. On it, Rogue teaches people how to turn their home into their own autonomous zones, or at least trend in that direction.

In May 2020, as protests heated up in Minneapolis, Portland, and Seattle, Rogue published a nine-minute video called "How to Survive Riots."[30] "Swiftly and fiercely, they have turned from peaceful protests to rioting and looting across the U.S.," Rogue said, wearing a cowboy hat.[31] "This is not fear-mongering. This is fact."[32]

Her first tip: "Steer clear of large cities. This is where these things are happening," adding, "in downtown, very large metropolitan cities."[33] Rogue long ago opted for the homestead life, living on forty acres with her husband, two daughters, and two dogs.

Her own homesteading adventures during the pandemic were challenged, as others crowded-in and built the skills they needed. Finding a sewing kit—the means of producing one's own clothes—proved difficult, Rogue said.[34]

"Sewing machines were never something I ever thought a pandemic of any kind would create a shortage of," Rogue said, during an August 2020 appearance on *The Safety Doc Podcast*. "People were realizing [the need for] a little more self-sufficiency."[35]

This increased effort toward achieving self-sufficiency extended past learning to sew and repair clothes to obtaining the most basic of necessities: food.

For Thine Own Self, Grow Food

If you cannot rely on the food system to deliver nourishment to your dinner table, nor rely on the government to protect home and hearth, or on schools to open their doors, it is on you to find those answers yourself. Homesteading is for people who want food they trust more than what exists at the grocery store. Canning is for people who do not trust the grocery store to keep its shelves stocked. Prepping is for people who believe a crisis is coming. It may not be imminent. But it is likely enough to plan for it. Homeschooling is for people who believe they can teach their kids better than the neighborhood school can.

Homeschoolers were a small minority of parents prior to the pandemic, but when schools kept their doors closed, parents turned their homes into schoolhouses. The U.S. Census Bureau reported that twice as many households were homeschooling at the start of the 2020–2021 school year than that at the start of 2019–2020.[36]

"It's clear that in an unprecedented environment, families are seeking solutions that will reliably meet their health and safety needs, their childcare needs, and the learning and socio-emotional needs of their children," commented Eggleston and Fields about the Census report.[37]

After the Y2K fiasco, when the computers did not melt down, and all that bottled water and box pasta was for naught, prepping took on a dim view in the public eye. As a *Vice* 2016 retrospective said: "The Y2K bug got the public more familiar with the survivalist lifestyle than ever. However, despite all the soothsayers warning the public to stock up for armageddon, the public didn't take the bait."[38]

The *Vice* story continued:

> A logical person could tell you that odds were high you were going to fall asleep as the ball dropped, wake up in the morning, turn on the lights, and still hear the dulcet tones of Moby's pop-electronica experiments rattling on the radio the next morning.
>
> But we weren't 100 percent sure, and it wasn't helped by the fact that the Y2K bug became a media craze in the years before we crossed the millennial finish line.[39]

When the lights never went out, preppers were considered along the lines of social hypochondriacs, as doomsdayers who seemed to hope for calamity as much as they predicted it.

But in 2020, when society's systems seemed shakier than ever, it was the prepper and the canner and the homeschooler who were vindicated.

For preppers, the "autonomous zones" that matter start within the mind and extend to the four walls of the home. At its most extreme, survivalism is not crowding in, it is opting-out from a world that no longer works as promised.

NOTES

1. Faith Popcorn. "Welcome to 2030: Come Cocoon With Me," Faith Popcorn's Brain Reserve (blog), June 15, 2020. https://faithpopcorn.com/trendblog/articles/post/welcome-to-2030/.

2. Popcorn, *Welcome to 2030*.

3. Ibid.

4. American Academy of Family Physicians (AAFP). "Seasonal Affective Disorder." *American Family Physician* 61, no. 5 (March 1, 2000): 1531–1532.

5. AAFP, *Seasonal Affective Disorder*, 1531–1532.

6. Mayo Clinic. "Seasonal Affective Disorder. Diagnosis and Treatment. Lifestyle and Home Remedies." Mayo Clinic. n.d. https://www.mayoclinic.org/diseases-conditions/seasonal-affective-disorder/diagnosis-treatment/drc-20364722.

7. Helliwell, John F., Richard Layard, Jeffrey Sachs, and Jan-Emmanuel De Neve, eds. 2021. "Happiness, Trust and Deaths under COVID-19. Figure 2.1: Ranking of Happiness 2018-2020." World Happiness Report 2021. Chapter 2, Page 20. March 20, 2021. https://worldhappiness.report/.

8. Clarke, Jodi. "Benefits of the Cozy Wellness Trend Hygge." Very Well Mind. June 27, 2021. https://www.verywellmind.com/health-benefits-of-hygge-4164281.

9. Parkinson, Justin. "Hygge: A Heart-Warming Lesson from Denmark." BBC News Magazine. October 2, 2015. https://www.bbc.com/news/magazine-34345791.

10. Hedgpeth, Dana. "So Many Pets Have Been Adopted During the Pandemic That Shelters Are Running Out." The Washington Post. January 6, 2021. https://www.washingtonpost.com/dc-md-va/2021/01/06/animal-shelters-coronavirus-pandemic/.

11. Arnold, Chris. "More Space, Please: Home Sales Booming Despite Pandemic, Recession." National Public Radio. August 28, 2020. https://www.npr.org/2020/08/28/906725372/more-space-please-home-sales-booming-despite-pandemic-recession.

12. Cramer, Maria and Aimee Ortiz. "They're Stuck at Home, So They're Making Home a Sanctuary." New York Times. September 4, 2020. https://www.nytimes.com/2020/09/04/business/coronavirus-home-upgrades.html.

13. Cramer and Ortiz, *They're Stuck at Home*.

14. Ibid.

15. Bodenheimer, Rebecca. "What's Behind the Pandemic Puzzle Craze?" JSTOR. December 16, 2020. https://daily.jstor.org/whats-behind-the-pandemic-puzzle-craze/.

16. Doubek, James and Art Silverman. "With People Stuck at Home, Jigsaw Puzzle Sales Soar." National Public Radio. April 13, 2020. https://www.npr.org/sections/coronavirus-live-updates/2020/04/13/833346707/with-people-stuck-at-home-jigsaw-puzzle-sales-soar.

17. Doubek and Silverman, *Jigsaw Puzzle Sales Soar*.

18. Snouwaert, Jessica. "10 Unlikely Items That Are Flying Off the Shelves During the Coronavirus Pandemic." Business Insider. April 26, 2020. https://www.businessinsider.com/coronavirus-sales-increases-unlikely-items-selling-well-high-demand-2020-4.

19. Jenkins, Craig. "All the Verzuz Battles, Ranked." Vulture.com. November 20, 2020. https://www.vulture.com/2020/11/verzuz-instagram-live-battles-ranked.html.

20. Jenkins, *All the Verzuz Battles, Ranked*.

21. Cramer and Ortiz, *They're Stuck at Home*.

22. Schwartz, Ian. "Seattle Mayor Durkan: CHAZ Has a 'Block Party Atmosphere,' Could Turn Into 'Summer of Love.'" Real Clear Politics. June 12, 2020. https://www.realclearpolitics.com/video/2020/06/12/seattle_mayor_durkan_chaz_has_a_block_party_atmosphere_could_turn_into_summer_of_love.html.

23. Schwartz, *Seattle Mayor Durkan.*

24. Abrams, Rachel. "Police Clear Seattle's Protest 'Autonomous Zone.'" The New York Times. July 1, 2020. https://www.nytimes.com/2020/07/01/us/seattle-protest-zone-CHOP-CHAZ-unrest.html.

25. Wall Street Journal Editorial Board. "Goodbye, Summer of Love." The Wall Street Journal. December 13, 2020. https://www.wsj.com/articles/goodbye-summer-of-love-11607898398.

26. Webber, Tammy and Sophia Tareen. "Unrest Emerges in Neighborhoods, Suburbs Beyond City Centers." The Associated Press. US News and World Report. July 1, 2020. https://www.usnews.com/news/us/articles/2020-06-01/unrest-emerges-in-neighborhoods-suburbs-beyond-city-centers.

27. Gray, Melissa. "All That Time in the Kitchen During This Pandemic Has Led to a Nationwide Shortage of Mason Jars." CNN. October 7, 2020. https://www.cnn.com/2020/10/07/us/mason-jars-canning-lids-shortage-trnd/index.html.

28. Morgan Rogue, "Survival Expert Morgan Rogue: Subtle Signs of Chaos." Interview by David P. Perrodin. *The Safety Doc Podcast*, August 7, 2020. https://www.youtube.com/watch?v=lcKSm-1n7Zc.

29. Rogue, *Survival Expert Morgan Rogue.*

30. Ibid.

31. Ibid.

32. Ibid.

33. Ibid.

34. Ibid.

35. Ibid.

36. Eggleston, Casey and Jason Fields. "Census Bureau's Household Pulse Survey Shows Significant Increase in Homeschooling Rates in Fall 2020." U.S. Census Bureau. March 22, 2021. https://www.census.gov/library/stories/2021/03/homeschooling-on-the-rise-during-covid-19-pandemic.html.

37. Eggleston and Fields, *Census Bureau's Household Pulse Survey.*

38. Smith, Ernie. "Canned Food, Doomsday Fears and the Y2K Hoarding Disaster That Didn't Happen." Vice. July 21, 2016. https://www.vice.com/en/article/bmvy8d/canned-food-doomsday-fears-and-the-y2k-hoarding-disaster-that-didnt-happen.

39. Smith, *Canned Food, Doomsday Fears.*

Chapter 6

The Continuum of Chaos

We generally perceive crisis events as a light switch: the time before the event, where the light is "on," and then after, as we are plunged into the darkness of uncertainty. Force majeures and black swan events thus fit neatly into our expectation bias toward understanding chaos. However, we will see that these on/off distinctions do not accurately or fully describe chaos events in real time. But first, we need to understand how binary thinking is applied to chaotic situations.

FORCE MAJEURES AND BLACK SWANS

Force Majeure is a French term meaning *superior force*. It is also a legal term of art referring to an "act of God." A party to a contract is not liable for a failure to perform if he can prove that (1) the failure was due to an impediment beyond his control; (2) he could not have reasonably foreseen the impediment at the time of contract formation; and (3) he could not have reasonably avoided or overcome its effects.

Evidence that force majeure are quasi-predictable events is that we have periodic tornado siren tests and Tsunami warning sirens. We do not know if or when these disasters will strike, but we know that they can and will happen and as such, we prepare for them. There is a measure of predictability with force majeure.

By contrast, a black swan is unforeseeable and changes the worldview. In the 1600s, scientists declared that swans were white. In 1697, Dutch navigator Willem de Vlamingh found black swans in Western Australia. [1] It shook everyone's confidence in "the system" and showed how risky it is to declare something impossible.

"A black swan is an unpredictable event that is beyond what is normally expected of a situation and has potentially severe consequences," writes Nassim Nicholas Taleb, a former Wall Street trader, in his book *The Black Swan: The Impact of the Highly Improbable*.[2] He continues, "Black swan events are characterised by their extreme rarity, their severe impact, and the widespread insistence they were obvious in hindsight."[3]

Force majeure and black swan both exceed what could reasonably be tolerated by a system. But unlike a force majeure, which is expected to be transitory, a black swan describes the implications of the event as it reshapes societal behaviors.

A force majeure event causes a restaurant to cobble together curbside delivery because its dining area will suddenly be closed for the next two weeks. The black swan occurrence spurs a new concept, the ghost kitchen that is specifically designed for the preparation of delivery-only meals. There is no storefront. There are no tables for customers.

Force majeure is a measure of magnitude. How much have things been disrupted and how soon can they return to normal? Black swan events are lasting in their effect on society. They are multigenerational. What has been permanently disrupted?

There are three examples of black swan events within recent history: the collapse of the Soviet Union, the terrorist attack on U.S. soil on September 11, 2001, and the COVID-19 pandemic.

For total control, you need a totalitarian state, a system the Soviet Union tried to build. Surrounded by capitalists on all sides, the narrative weaved by men no one in the country ever heard of, told a story of a world hostile to Communism, waiting to pounce and crush the young, progressive nation on its mission to unshackle the planet from the slavery of exploitation. Everyone wants to see us fail, the narrative suggested. Or dead. Death is better. Death is forever.

What follows is a recollection of history that led up and contributed to the esca-
lation of the Chernobyl disaster and demise of the Soviet Union as experienced
directly by Nikolai Razouvaev, the Soviet-born competitive long-distance cyclist
who was a member of the Soviet National Cycling Team between 1984–1990,
and who is fluent in the historical chronicles of his native country.[4]

On June 22, 1941, an enemy the Soviet Union had previously made peace with attacked with vicious force. The Germans went all in on Operation Barbarossa to wipe the Soviets from the world's scene. *Wehrmacht* outnumbered the Red Army on all counts; tanks, airplanes, men, guns, and munitions.

No one in the Union of Soviet Socialist Republics (USSR) expected Germany to attack. Five months later, the Nazis stood 25 kilometers from

Moscow's outskirts ready to devour our capital. We were taught that we were a peaceful nation attacked by capitalist monsters. We were taught we won because, despite looking weak and being outmanned and outgunned, we had faith in the communist way, which would save us all.

Today, with some archives opened to researchers, it looks like the Soviets outnumbered the Germans by four tanks to one, had three times as many planes and almost double the guns and mortars.[5] Messaging from shadowy sources triumphed over truth.

The Red Army had the hardware but not the will to fight for a political ideology that men its generals and soldiers never heard of suggested they should believe in. What the soldiers saw with their own eyes—fathers, brothers, neighbors taken away in handcuffs, never to return, never to be seen again, millions of people dying of hunger in lands rich in produce—did not match the official prosperity and progress narrative flowing out from the storytellers.

Twenty-four years after the Great October Revolution, people began to doubt the story; people asked themselves why the narrative feels made up, why it feels fake. The soldiers had nothing to fight for and without an ideation worth dying for, they raised their arms up and surrendered.

That is how the Germans sliced the Red Army to pieces and came up to Moscow's backyard. The story, the narrative meant to unite everyone, failed its goal. Skepticism reigned, faith in the idea died.

The problem with fake narratives is that it is hard to make the populace play along if no one believes the story. You can force it down their throats, make everyone follow the script, but turning the screws too far brings bloodshed with it, death and suffering people never forget.

When Mikhail Gorbachev seized power over the Communist Party in 1985, everyone born in the 1950s and later lived, their thinking shaped by the narrative dictated by shadowy, unknown men. Rumors of Stalin's killings were billed as collateral damage and the necessary means to establish order in a traditionally disorderly, chaotic country. They were heroic, against the odds, and yet were still victorious in the Great Patriotic War, and had now reached the rebuilding stage on the road to communist nirvana.

The new general secretary did what no other Soviet leader before him dared to do—unlock the door to the Soviet Union's dark and bloody past. He allowed previously hidden, secret material to tear through people's minds with stories of horror and atrocities carried out by the state against its citizens. He borrowed a word from Lenin and called the opened floodgates to classified information *Glasnost* (openness), a bold suggestion that the radical new path he wanted to take the country with him on will be a game changer.

It looked and felt like he meant business. The Soviet news outlets, dominated by four central Moscow-based newspapers sunk in a sea of new, independent periodicals publishing everything from gossip and alien invasion rumors to detailed accounts of the Bolshevik coup, Stalin's purges, and corruption reports on past political leaders.

They left the narrative's core intact—the Party's benevolence and good will was evidenced by *Glasnost*, sealed by confessions of past sins, and publicized repentance for the evil deeds no one living now should be held responsible for. What's past is past. Keep reading, keep marveling, and stay amazed. We have new things waiting for you, let us do our job.

Then, Chernobyl blew up, and the carefully crafted narratives began to blow up, also. Unrest and political conflict began to crescendo toward the official dissolution of the USSR in 1991. Ongoing conflict between former Soviet republics continues to the present day.

Another black swan event began the moment that first plane struck the first World Trade Center Tower. Killing thousands and forever burned into the collective consciousness of all Americans, the terrorist attack on 9/11 ushered in the Patriot Act and the idea of (further) government encroachment into personal privacy for the sake of public safety. The 9/11 attack also brought the United States down the path of war with Iraq over alleged weapons of mass destruction (WMD). The changes brought about by the tragedy have had, and will continue to have, long-lasting impacts on American society, both from a psychological standpoint and a very real physical standpoint through increased governmental regulation. In fact, some of the freedoms given up in the name of public safety after 9/11 paved the way for additional loss of freedom during the pandemic.

The COVID-19 black swan changed so much for so many. Governmental lockdowns created tertiary problems, including higher rates of depression and suicide, unemployment, and food insecurity.[6] The consequences from the approach to control the spread of the virus have had far-ranging impacts.

For example, consequences from the pandemic now factor into the decision-making for people's career choices (e.g., Essential vs. Nonessential). In Seattle, realtors can no longer sell studios and one bedrooms as people now want a home-office option, so it is affecting the real estate market.

Stacey Brower had worked in the Seattle, Washington real estate market for fourteen years before witnessing the effects of the COVID-19 black swan.

Housing in Seattle was limited and expensive prior to COVID-19. Following the pandemic lockdowns there was an exodus from downtown condos and apartments to the suburbs. People no longer had to commute and wanted more space for home offices and yards. They were less willing to tolerate high rents and many buildings only allowed one to two people per elevator so using the elevator became time consuming as well as a potential health risk. With the downtown restaurants, parks and stores being closed the benefits of living downtown dwindled.[7]

Whether the effects on the real estate market from COVID-19 may be permanent due to changes in the workforce's ability to work remotely will ultimately describe the extent of that black swan event.

In each of the three examples, the black swan events were not predictable and had far-reaching, long-term impact on affected society. These are critical distinctions from force majeure events such as a hurricane crisscrossing the Caribbean. Distinguishing the difference between force majeure and black swan events is somewhat analogous to the difference between crisis and chaos, as we will see.

CRISIS OR CHAOS

Crisis implies a decisive point in a dangerous situation with anticipation of an abrupt change to the condition, for better or for worse. A crisis may be characterized by a bifurcation, which is a parameter-dependent change in dynamical behavior. A useful distinction exists between hard (abrupt) and soft (gradual) bifurcations.

Hard bifurcation: the ice on a lake slowly warms (temperature is the bifurcation parameter) and suddenly breaks, dropping you into the cold lake.

Soft bifurcation: an ice cube (temperature is again the bifurcation parameter) once at a temperature greater than or equal to 32 degrees slowly melts into a glass of Scotch.

A soft bifurcation is clearly preferable, particularly because its impacts are dispersed over time.

As mathematically defined, a crisis occurs with the appearance of a strange attractor. The word "attractor" has nothing to do with gravitation. As in dynamic systems, attractors provide a way to describe the asymptotic behavior of typical orbits.

Operationally, this means that there is a dramatic change in the dynamical behavior of the system. The present disconnects from the past and the past behavior has little or no predictive value as the system navigates its way through a profoundly altered landscape.

In a fiat money economy, sudden-onset hyperinflation might be characterized as a strange attractor resulting in extraordinary behaviors in the country's monetary system. For example, during the 1923 hyperinflation crisis of the Weimar Republic, "workers were often paid twice per day because prices rose so fast their wages were virtually worthless by lunc htime."[8]

In addition, "[f]armers refused to take any form of paper money for their crops. The harvest of 1923 sat in farmers' warehouses while supermarkets in the cities were empty. Starvation and civil unrest loomed."[9]

The more interesting question is what happened next. What was the shape of the dynamical trajectory as the economic crisis resolved?

A crisis is often of short duration and will have an identifiable turning point(s). It tends to scale in a predictable manner. People believe their own actions might resolve a crisis. Because a crisis has a degree of certainty, responses to it can be scripted and practiced, such as a fire drill or contingency planning for a looming workers strike.

The New York City transit strike of 2005 is an example of a crisis. Contract negotiations reached an impasse (hard bifurcation) and at 3:00 a.m. on December 20, 2005, transit workers walked off their jobs, bringing a halt to the mass transit system in America's biggest city. Around 6,000 subway cars and 4,500 buses were idled.[10]

The strike tossed a wrench into the plans of millions of city residents, but also was not completely unexpected: prior transit and sanitation strikes had been resolved at the bargaining table. Due to its unpopularity, the strike ended on December 23, 2005.[11]

An unresolved crisis might become an emergency that could, in turn, change into a chaos situation which could affect an individual, group, community, or population. An example of a crisis that could have turned to chaos is if there had been an escalation to the use of nuclear weapons during the 1962 Cuban Missile Crisis.

Chaos is a state of disorder that is amorphous and without clear turning points. Chaos quickly or gradually settles into outcome basins or creates a new mean. Chaos describes a system that will develop in unpredictable ways and will not scale linearly. It exists on a continuum with degrees of absorption by systems. A state of chaos, due to a lack of, or impossibility of, a scripted response will usually, if not inevitably, spread. Chaos affects the global consciousness, even if only temporarily.

As chaos is uncertain, people do not feel that their actions will resolve it, but rather that they might be able to change their behaviors to better adjust to the situation. The nonlinear features of chaos present significant challenges to routine-seeking people who must overcome habitual behavior in order to adapt their patterns to evolving network conditions.

For example, modern-day emergency managers do not conduct nuclear missile attack drills in major American cities, in part, due to the unlikelihood of such events and also due to the incalculable cascade effect of compounding consequences.

An interesting feature about chaotic systems that warrants emphasis is that they can exhibit very orderly behavior for long periods of time before making an abrupt transition even though the attractor topology has not changed (in contrast with a bifurcation).

Consider the Rössler attractor in mathematical differential equations. It can spend a prolonged time in a near-periodic orbit on the *xy*-lane and then make an abrupt transition on the *z*-axis.

In other words, when chaos occurs for long periods of times, humans might perceive that it has reached a steady state, or a new familiar and predictable torus, as described in part 1 of this book when it was noted that humans seek routines and patterns in their lives. But the Rössler attractor demonstrates that the mere perception of a steady state does not necessarily mean a steady state has been achieved.

Thus, while chaos is generally believed to be binary, either there is chaos or there is not, as we will see, there are actually four states of chaos.

BRIEF AND LOCALIZED CHAOS (1–5 DAYS): CERTAINTY

The first state of chaos is characterized by the limited nature of three conditions:

- **Duration:** The event has a short temporal duration.
- **Localization:** The event is autonomous to the area with negligible spill over to other proximal locations or networks.
- **Recovery:** A brief and localized event has minimal effect on the day-to-day lives of people outside the area where this event happens. It is unlikely to have long-lasting negative impacts, and the life span of its aftereffects is short.

Examples of brief and localized chaos events include the 2007 I-35W Mississippi River bridge collapse and the 2020 Salt Lake County, Utah earthquake.

The Interstate 35W bridge disaster in Minneapolis killed 13 people and injured 145 when the bridge broke apart due to a structural failure during rush hour on August 1, 2007.[12] The catastrophe disrupted emergency services, Mississippi river and land transit, and cellular communication networks in and around Minnesota's biggest city. Subsequently, Minneapolis expended resources to restore emergency, transportation, and communication services to the area.

In Utah, "Salt Lake County's March 18, 2020 earthquake, whose epicenter was near downtown, damaged well over 160 historic buildings and left several unfit for human occupation at least for a short while."[13] Structural engineers and government inspectors assessed the integrity of natural gas lines, transportation infrastructure, and buildings over the next few days—and did so in a county of 1.1 million people who were only two weeks into a COVID-19 stay home decree.[14]

Although damage was modest, there was a heightened possibility for additional seismic activity. Eight hours after the earthquake, the U.S. Geological Survey posted on Twitter, "The chance of an earthquake of magnitude 3 or higher is 90%, and it is likely that as few as 0 or as many as 220 such earthquakes may occur in the case that the sequence is re-invigorated by a larger aftershock."[15]

Luckily, there were no significant aftershocks in Salt Lake County to prolong the chaos, and the emergency situation caused by the collapsed bridge in Minnesota was resolved within a relatively short time frame. Therefore, both events were brief and localized.

INTERMEDIATE AND REGIONAL CHAOS
(6–90 DAYS): MODERATE CERTAINTY

In this state of chaos, the impacted area is regional. It is intermediate with more lasting effects as more systems break down over time. Chaos intensifies for this reason as other systems are impacted. There is a cascade effect.

Loss of continuity in systems of food distribution, transport, and energy supply leads to secondary problems as hygiene starts to break down, which can then cause cholera outbreaks. Loss of life may or may not be higher than other chaos states, but fatalities are spread out over a longer period of time. Anticipate finite voltage effect at the population level.

There is an incremental, prioritized re-start of systems. Assets will be prioritized, and it might take several days or weeks to return to pre-event levels of operation. People view the event as *very likely* to be transitory.

Examples of intermediate and regional chaos events include the European heat wave of 2003 and the 2021 Colonial Pipeline Ransomware Attack.

Following a hot and dry July, from August 1 to 20, 2003, Europe experienced an historic heat wave that killed an estimated 15,000 people.[16] In London, trains were shut down over fears that tracks would buckle in the heat. Throughout France, Spain, Portugal, and Italy, the intense heat and dry conditions sparked devastating forest fires.[17]

With French river temperatures hitting record highs, nuclear power plants that relied on river water cooling were forced to scale back electricity generation, both for domestic use and export, just as millions of people were glued to their air conditioning units.[18] The region idled for a month as people limited their exposure to the outdoors to prevent heat-related illness. However, as dire as conditions became, Europeans knew this heat event would terminate at some point when the weather inevitably transitioned to winter.

On May 6, 2021, a cybercriminal organization known only as Darkside hacked into the computer network of the Colonial Pipeline Company.[19] "The operator took itself offline the next day and shut key conduits delivering 45% of the [United States'] East Coast's supply of diesel, petrol and jet fuel."[20]

The supply crunch sparked panic-buying in the U.S. Southeast, bringing long lines and high prices at gas stations just ahead of the peak summer driving season. North Carolina issued a State of Emergency and "more than 1,000 gas stations in the Southeast reported running out of fuel."[21]

Colonial paid the four-million-dollar ransom demanded by Darkside and incrementally restarted fuel distribution on May 12.[22] Lower priority nodes (less dense population areas) were not fully replenished with fuel supplies for another ten to fourteen days due to a combination of technical problems in fuel orders and ongoing panic-buying and hoarding by consumers.

In both cases, the effects of the heatwave and ransomware attack were regional and caused additional cascading effects. But there still existed a sense that these events were finite and could be resolved given enough time. But what happens when the chaos event lasts longer?

EXTENDED AND INTERNATIONAL CHAOS (90 DAYS TO INDETERMINATE DURATION): UNCERTAINTY

This stage of chaos creates uncertainty as to when, or if, it will end. Anticipate crowd-in behavior as people retreat from stressful situations. There is no idea of how it will scale. There are no tested protocols to implement to resolve the condition. No population-level rehearsal. It requires developing mitigating measures in the moment that might provide relief for a day or two.

Simulated annealing occurs as governments progressively assess options and make choices to arrive at a more desirable outcome basin. This cycle happens over and over as governments attempt to handle an extended chaos situation.

These types of events may require an international response; national borders are not relevant. As Nikolai Razouvaev shared in part 2, airborne radioactive isotopes spewing from Chernobyl did not respect property lines. At this level, it will be impossible to determine the long-term effects of the actual event itself.

There are also multigenerational effects. This type of chaos situation changes behaviors beyond the generation that is immediately affected—a generation beyond the people who experienced it in real time. For example, children born to parents who survived the Great Depression may re-use aluminum foil, keep and repurpose everything, and maintain a secondary pantry.

Examples of extended and international chaos events include World War II (1939–1945) and the 1986 Chernobyl nuclear reactor fire.

Between the years 1939–1945, virtually every part of the world was involved in the war fought between the Axis Powers (Germany, Italy, and Japan) and the Allied Powers (Britain, the United States, the Soviet Union, and France). The statistics on World War II casualties are inexact. Worldwide casualties are estimated at fifteen million battle deaths, twenty-five million battle wounded, and forty-five million civilian deaths.[23] About 3 percent of the entire world's population died during the war.

While the war waged, major uncertainty existed as to whether the war would ever end. Governments on both sides repeatedly changed strategies, both on the battlefield and at home, to attempt to adapt to ongoing chaos. The generational impact of the multiyear war has been massive and ongoing.

With similar impact, on April 25, 1986, the worst nuclear accident in history unfolded near the city of Chernobyl in the former USSR. The fire burned for ten days, releasing a large amount of radionuclides into the atmosphere, affecting much of Europe and bringing great concern for radioactive contamination across the globe.[24]

In the months following the accident, millions of people living in northern USSR and Western Europe braced for food instability or radiation-caused illness or death. "Persistent myths and misperceptions about the threat of radiation have resulted in 'paralyzing fatalism' among residents of affected areas."[25] The environmental and regulatory impacts of the Chernobyl accident persist to the present day.

World War II and the Chernobyl incident both illustrate the long-term effects of extended and international chaos. What if either of these events had been compounded by another event? The fourth state of chaos occurs when a secondary event happens in conjunction with an extended and international event.

COMORBID CHAOS (INDETERMINATE DURATION): UNCERTAINTY

This fourth state of chaos includes qualities of Extended and International chaos events with the addition of one or more secondary, population-level chaos events that are intermediate and regional or extended and international. The secondary event happens concurrently with some or the entire primary event.

In addition, chaos at this level oscillates in intensity. For example, there may be civil unrest affected by weather patterns (e.g., protests taper off on rainy days). Populations exhibit a lack of trust in government and authority. There is a corresponding loss of credibility by those in authority due to changing narratives.

Examples of comorbid chaos include The Great Depression from 1929 to 1939 confounded by the 1931–1939 Great Plains Dust Bowl and the 2020 COVID-19 pandemic in conjunction with racial justice protests.

The Great Depression was the worst economic downturn in the history of the industrialized world, lasting from 1929 to 1939.[26] In 1932, many politicians, businessmen, and journalists started to contemplate the possibility of massive revolution in the United States. In fact, thousands of the most desperate unemployed workers began raiding food stores.[27]

At the store, the price of chicken fell from 38 cents a pound to 12 cents, the price of eggs dropped from 50 cents a dozen to just over 13 cents, and the price of gasoline fell from 10 cents a gallon to less than a nickel. Still, many families went hungry, and few could afford to own a car.[28]

By 1933, when the Great Depression reached its lowest point, some fifteen million Americans were unemployed and nearly half the country's banks had failed.[29]

Economic stability gradually returned in 1939 due, in part, to government New Deal projects that reformed financial systems and put people back to work. Many people who lived through the era distrusted banks and would no longer buy goods using credit.

But before the economic improvement, the Dust Bowl intensified the crushing economic impacts of the Great Depression. In 1931, severe drought hit the Midwestern and Southern Plains of the United States. As crops died, crumbling topsoil from over-plowed and over-grazed land led to powerful dust storms that pummeled the region.[30] "Residents crawled to safety in the dust (summer) storms and 'snust' (winter) storms. Many towns were abandoned."[31]

Hundreds of people succumbed to what doctors at the time called "dust pneumonia," a respiratory illness caused by tiny inorganic particles in the windblown dust.[32] Famine gripped the region as it was impossible to sustain livestock. "Cattle went blind and suffocated. When farmers cut them open, they found stomachs stuffed with fine sand."[33]

In the fall of 1939, rain finally returned in significant amounts to many areas of the Great Plains, signaling the end of the Dust Bowl. The positive weather change coincided with economic recovery stimulated by the New Deal to bring relief to millions of Americans.

Another comorbid chaos event surfaced more recently. "In late December 2019, an outbreak of a mysterious pneumonia characterized by fever, dry cough, and fatigue, and occasional gastrointestinal symptoms happened in a seafood wholesale wet market, the Huanan Seafood Wholesale Market, in Wuhan, Hubei, China."[34] Little did the world suspect that what was happening in China was a forecast of what would happen the world over.

On January 31, 2020, the World Health Organization (WHO) issued a Global Health Emergency for just the sixth time in its seventy-one years of existence as human-to-human transmission of the novel coronavirus disease (COVID-19) was quickly spreading across the United States, Germany, Japan, Vietnam, and Taiwan.[35] Billions of people were ordered to stay in their homes.

The COVID-19 pandemic led to a dramatic loss of human life worldwide and presented extraordinary challenges to public health, food systems, and employment. Vaccine rollouts in early 2021 were credited with dramatically reducing cases of COVID-19.

The pandemic was the catalyst for rapid adoption of telemedicine, remote work, and distance learning. The pandemic-driven social constructs of essential and nonessential workers will influence career choices for years to come.

The summer of 2020 also saw the United States' biggest protests for racial justice and civil rights in a generation. "Despite a worsening COVID-19 pandemic, tens of thousands took to the streets to demand change—first in Minneapolis, and later in New York, Washington, Portland, and elsewhere."[36]

Anti-racism demonstrators also marched to show their support in cities overseas including Brussels and London. "Despite the media focus on looting and vandalism, however, there is little evidence to suggest that demonstrators have engaged in widespread violence."[37] Regardless, the perception of violence persisted, and many questioned the safety and advisability of mass public gatherings for demonstrations during a pandemic.

As noted, chaos is not a binary event. Nor does chaos require temporal or geographic confinement. Certainty of duration and extent plays a significant role in determining which level of chaos state exists along a continuum. These factors make the difference in individual and population-level perception of chaos, such as the difference between a bridge collapse and a world war, or a pandemic confounded by additional chaos events.

THE VELOCITY OF INFORMATION IN 2020

The velocity of information in the year 2020 is depicted in the following four figures. Joined together, they create a longitudinal mosaic of the constructs of velocity of information, black swan, finite voltage, wet bulb, crowd-in behavior, and regression to the mean as they appeared on the timeline of 2020 (figures 6.1–6.4).

These themes were explained in previous chapters and the purpose of incorporating them into figures is to display subtle trends and patterns of relationship, as well as to communicate processes that are easier to identify on a timeline.

VELOCITY OF INFORMATION
David P. Perrodin, PhD

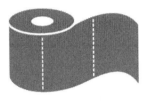

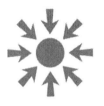

Scarcity Mindset
* Binge buy toilet paper, sanitizers, soup, pasta...

Availability Cascade
* Self-reinforcing public discourse

Scatter information "Ventilators"

Increased velocity of information toward us - emails from companies, local news covering local stories

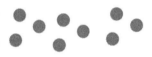

MARCH 13, 2020

END OF MARCH 2020

REMEMBER AS UTOPIA

SENSE OF EXCITEMENT

BLACK SWAN
* Onset of chaos
    Δ from Torus
    * Predictable day-to-day similarity rapidly displaced by uncertainty
* Cognitive dissonance
    * Forced compliance
    * New information

Figure 6.1   Velocity of Info—Onset of Chaos—March 2020. *Credit David P. Perrodin and Aimee K. DiStefano;* Figure by David P. Perrodin and Aimee K. DiStefano. Image use granted by Pixabay license. Free for commercial use, no attribution required. Toilet paper image #6278416 by chiplaney from Pixabay. https://pixabay.com/illustrations/toilet-paper -roll-vintage-retro-6278416/.

Note: The COVID-19 pandemic was a black swan event. Humans experienced an abrupt change from their predictable routines and day-to-day similarity was displaced by uncertainty. People initially felt excited by the newness of the pandemic. Scarcity mindset prompted binge purchasing of necessities as people were panicked by scatter information (numbers, buzz words, and opinions) haphazardly tossed into communication streams by news media attempting to be first instead of being accurate. Previously unfamiliar words such as "ventilators" and "coronavirus" were commonplace in rushed news reports. People grasped and recited available information, leading to self-reinforcing public discourse of dire scenarios. The velocity of information was calibrated directly to individuals in late March as companies emailed their consumers statements of solidarity and support and local news media broke from repeating national scripts to cover local news stories of the pandemic's impacts proximal to the viewer.

PANDEMIC / CIVIL UNREST

<u>New Vocab</u>
- Social Distance
- Essential Worker
- Safer at Home
- Flatten the Curve
- Contact Tracing
- Self-quarantine

Civilians languishing, anger,
depression, anxiety

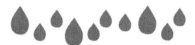

"Wet bulb" effect - unable
to escape density of negative
information atmosphere

MAY/JUNE/JULY
2020

<u>Finite Voltage</u> (~90 days)
"Breaking point for civilian
population"

"Mental burnout"

HEALTH CARE HEROES PARADES

APRIL-MAY

PERMANENT TECHNOLOGY SHIFTS

- Remote workplace
- Remote learning
- Telemedicine
- Online shopping, curbside pickup

(TIME DILATION EFFECT - Greatest Impact on Children)

Figure 6.2   Velocity of Info—Finite Voltage— April, May, June, July 2020. *Credit David P. Perrodin and Aimee K. DiStefano;* Figure by David P. Perrodin and Aimee K. DiStefano.

Note: As the COVID-19 pandemic approached ninety days, civilian populations experienced finite voltage, or reached their breaking point. This breakage was characterized by languishing, anxiety, anger, and depression. Media coverage centered on negative pandemic and social unrest stories and messaging reinforced the uncertainty to create a "wet bulb" environment in which it became difficult for individuals to escape gloomy information as they went about their daily activities. New vocabulary terms, such as *flatten the curve* and *social distancing*, took root into our everyday communication. Morale-boosting events, including healthcare heroes parades, were intended to increase resiliency to finite voltage. The disrupting features of the black swan event ushered in permanent technology shifts including remote work, telemedicine, distance learning, and online shopping.

FAILURE to REGRESS to the MEAN

- fatigue of just-in-time manufacturing systems -

COIN SHORTAGE

- slowing of in-person commerce -

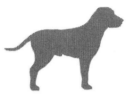

Surround self with comfort items: puzzles, games, pillows, outdoor pools, interior paint, pets

Spend less on scarcity items

New vocabulary becomes part of our lexicons
- In 2017, it was "spaghetti map" for hurricane paths
- In 2020, fifteen new terms! *(this is a lot for humans to process)*

AUGUST 2020

SEPTEMBER/ OCTOBER 2020

Crowd-In Behavior
Civilians expect to be in chaos for months or years - no definite end point
- Fading belief that this is a transitory period
- Plant food gardens, canning supplies, freezers

Disrupting Finite Voltage
1. Embrace Crowd-in
2. "I observed"
3. Name your fears
4. Talk to yourself in the third person
5. Parkinson's Law
   - Restore start and end routines of workday
6. Change things every 60 days
7. Expressive writing or create art
8. Spend more time outdoors
9. Exercise

Figure 6.3 Velocity of Info—Crowd-in Behavior August, September, October 2020. *Credit David P. Perrodin and Aimee K. DiStefano;* Figure by David P. Perrodin and Aimee K. DiStefano. Image use granted by Pixabay license. Free for commercial use, no attribution required. Dog silhouette image #5890164 by Please Don't sell My Artwork AS IS from Pixabay. https://pixabay.com/vectors/dog-animal-silhouette-5890164/

Note: Approximately four months into the chaos event, population-level behavior shifted from scarcity buying and languishing to a *crowd-in* mindset. The chaotic situation changed, but did not subside. There was no regression to the mean, or return to typical daily life prior to the onset of the chaos event. Civilians expected to be in chaos for months or years and that there was no definite end-point to the current condition. It was not transitory, like a heat spell in a cold weather climate. New vocabulary words, such as *social distance*, evolved into our daily lexicons. We fluently incorporated the words into our regular communications and abided by their actionable meanings. Social distance meant to stand 6 feet away from another person. Realizing the limitations of in-person activities, people acquired items that made them feel comfortable in their homes. These items included puzzles, games, pillows, outdoor pools, and pets. To stave off finite voltage, people deployed strategies to help them feel that they had control over the situations and experiences that affected their lives. Restoring start and end routines to their workdays, exercise, and using the words "I observed" were all techniques to overlay control and cope with stress during a prolonged chaos event.

Democratic Party wins
Presidential Election
- Media coverage of politics,
  civil unrest, COVID-19,
  and economy shift to
  positive framing

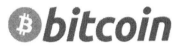

Record highs for stock market
and Bitcoin
- Miles long lines at food
  banks

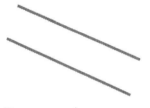

Sharp regression
toward the mean

Wall Street - Main Street
disconnect

OPTIMISM FOR "RETURN TO NORMAL"

NOVEMBER/DECEMBER
2020

Revised Social Contract
- Large scale acceptance of
  censorship by media and
  corporations to reduce
  alleged misinformation
  - Corporate and
    individual social
    credit scores
- Contemplation of truth
  and reconciliation

Compliance Behavior
- Increased COVID-19
  restrictions
- Cancel holiday gatherings
  - Backlash
- Peltzman Effect
  - Riskier behavior due to
    imminent vaccine and
    anticipated government
    stimulus money
    - Mask becomes
      fashion accessory

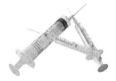

Figure 6.4 Velocity of Info—Regression to the Mean—November, December 2020.
Credit David P. Perrodin and Aimee K. DiStefano; Figure by David P. Perrodin and Aimee K. DiStefano. Images use granted by Pixabay license. Free for commercial use, no attribution required. Syringe image #5029289 by ds_30 from Pixabay and scales image #36417 by Clicker-Free-Vector Images from Pixabay. https://pixabay.com/vectors/scales-balance -symbol-justice-36417/. https://pixabay.com/photos/medical-white-isolated-medicine -5029289/. Bitcoin logo is in the public domain. https://commons.wikimedia.org/wiki/ File:Bitcoin_logo.svg.

Note: Previously negative media coverage of politics, civil unrest, COVID-19, and the economy promptly shifted to positive framing following the Democratic Party victory in the U.S. presidential election. COVID-19 vaccines received emergency use authorization and rollout programs were underway across the world. Population-level messaging communicated that everyday life would return to normal in 2021. People relaxed their crowd-in behavior. However, skepticism about the validity of the presidential election and questions about the safety of the vaccines were met with the apparent tightening censorship of citizens by government, media, and corporations. Governments also maintained, or even enhanced, restrictions on social gatherings, due to concerns that premature re-opening of businesses and venues might undermine the efforts to achieve herd immunity against COVID-19 or its variants. Compliance behavior was both authentic and feigned at a population level.

NOTES

1. Lowe, Tim. "Black Swan: The Impossible Bird." Australian Geographic. July 11, 2016. https://www.australiangeographic.com.au/topics/wildlife/2016/07/black-swan-the-impossible-bird/.

2. Taleb, Nassim Nicholas. *The Black Swan, Second Edition: The Impact of the Highly Improbable*, 2nd Edition Audio (New York: Random House Publishing Group, 2010).

3. Taleb, *The Black Swan*, 2nd Edition.

4. Nikolai Razouvaev, personal communications with the author, January 2021 to April 2021.

5. Meltyukhov, Mikhail Ivanovich. "Stalin's Missed Chance. The Soviet Union and the Struggle for Europe: 1939–1941." 2000. http://militera.lib.ru/research/meltyukhov/index.html. Author's Note: Soviet archives are often incomplete, inaccessible, and translated with varying levels of clarity, so exact figures are difficult to ascertain. During Soviet times of *samizdat*, accurate historical information was both produced infrequently and difficult to obtain or access.

6. Banerjee, Debanjan, Jagannatha Rao Kosagisharaf, and T.S. Sathyanarayana Rao. "'The Dual Pandemic' of Suicide and COVID-19: A Biopsychosocial Narrative of Risks and Preventions." Psychiatry Research, 295:113577. November 13, 2020. 3, Table 2 "Proposed risk factors and contributors for suicide during pandemics." 10.1016/j.psychres.2020.113577.

7. Stacey Brower, personal communication with the author, June 30, 2021.

8. BBC. "Bitesize The Weimar Republic 1918-1929: The Hyperinflation Crisis, 1923." https://www.bbc.co.uk/bitesize/guides/z9y64j6/revision/5.

9. Forbes. "In Hyperinflation's Aftermath, How Germany Went Back to Gold." Forbes.com. June 9, 2011. https://www.forbes.com/2011/06/09/germany-gold-standard.html?sh=330426c35934.

10. New York City Department of Transportation. "2005 Transit Strike: Transportation Impacts and Analysis." New York City. February 2006, 4. https://www1.nyc.gov/html/dot/downloads/pdf/transitstrike-1.pdf.

11. Solomon, Nancy. "New York City Buses, Subways Back on Track." National Public Radio (NPR)—All Things Considered [Transcription.] December 23, 2005. https://www.npr.org/templates/story/story.php?storyId=5068181.

12. MPR News Staff. "Photos: Looking Back at the I-35W Bridge Collapse." MPRNews. August 1, 2017. https://www.mprnews.org/story/2017/08/01/looking-back-photos-of-the-bridge-collapse.

13. Merritt, Christopher W. "Utah's Biggest Earthquake in History: And You Don't Even Probably Know About It." Utah Division of State History. April 3, 2020. https://history.utah.gov/utahs-biggest-earthquake-in-history-and-you-dont-even-probably-know-about-it-2/.

14. United States Census Bureau. "Population Estimates, July 1, 2019. Quick Facts. Salt Lake County, Utah." United States Census Bureau. 2021. https://www.census.gov/quickfacts/fact/table/saltlakecountyutah,UT/PST045219.

15. Becker, Andrew. "A 5.7 Magnitude Quake Shakes Utah, Largest Since 1992." KUER. March 18, 2020. https://www.kuer.org/news/2020-03-18/5-7-magnitude -quake-shakes-utah-largest-since-1992.

16. Fouillet, Anne, Grégoire Rey, Françoise Laurent, Gérard Pavillon, Stéphanie Bellec, Chantal Guihenneuc-Jouyeux, Jaceuline Clavel, Eric Jougla and Denis Hémon. "Excess Mortality Related to the August 2003 Heat Wave in France." *International Archives of Occupational and Environmental Health* 80, no. 1 (2006):16–24. doi: 10.1007/s00420-006-0089-4.

17. National Aeronautics and Space Administration. "European Heat Wave." Earth Observatory. 2021. https://earthobservatory.nasa.gov/images/3714/european -heat-wave.

18. The Guardian. "Heatwave Hits French Power Production." August 12, 2003. https://www.theguardian.com/world/2003/aug/12/france.nuclear.

19. Russon, Mary-Ann. "US Fuel Pipeline Hackers 'Didn't Mean to Create Problems.'" BBC News. May 10, 2021. https://www.bbc.com/news/business-57050690.

20. Russon, *US Fuel Pipeline Hackers.*

21. WSOC-TV News Staff. "'Panic-Buying' Leaving Gas Stations Dry Amid Colonial Pipeline Shutdown." WSCOTV. May 12, 2021. https://www.wsoctv.com/ news/local/some-local-gas-stations-see-shortages-amid-colonial-pipeline-shutdown/ XK3MT7Z4KZHQDKZHMLQOSCEECE/.

22. Kelly, Mary Louise, Jason Fuller and Justin Kenin. "The Colonial Pipeline CEO Explains The Decision To Pay Hackers A \$4.4 Million Ransom." All Things Considered, NPR. June 3, 2021. https://www.npr.org/2021/06/03/1003020300/colo-nial-pipeline-ceo-explains-the-decision-to-pay-hackers-4-4-million-ransom.

23. The National World War II Museum. "Research Starters: Worldwide Deaths in World War II." Worldwide Casualties. The National World War II Museum, New Orleans. 2021. https://www.nationalww2museum.org/students-teachers/student -resources/research-starters/research-starters-worldwide-deaths-world-war.

24. Blakemore, Erin. "The Chernobyl Disaster: What Happened, and the Long-Term Impacts." National Geographic. May 17, 2019. https://www.nationalgeographic .com/culture/article/chernobyl-disaster.

25. World Health Organization. "Chernobyl: The True Scale of the Accident. 20 Years Later a UN Report Provides Definitive Answers and Ways to Repair Lives." World Health Organization. September 5, 2005. https://www.who.int/news/item/05 -09-2005-chernobyl-the-true-scale-of-the-accident.

26. History.com Editors. "Great Depression History." History.com. October 29, 2009. https://www.history.com/topics/great-depression/great-depression-history.

27. Marx, Jerry D. "American Social Policy in the Great Depression and World War II." VCU Libraries Social Welfare History Project. 2011. http://socialwelfare .library.vcu.edu/eras/great-depression/american-social-policy-in-the-great-depres-sion-and-wwii.

28. Wheelock, David C. "The Great Depression: An Overview." Federal Reserve Bank of St. Louis. n.d.: 1. https://www.stlouisfed.org/~/media/files/pdfs/great-depres-sion/the-great-depression-wheelock-overview.pdf.

29. History.com Editors, *Great Depression History.*

30. American Experience. "Surviving the Dust Bowl. Timeline: The Dust Bowl." PBS. n.d. https://www.pbs.org/wgbh/americanexperience/features/dust-bowl-surviving-dust-bowl/.

31. Gordon, Dan. "When Deadly Dirt Devastated the Southern Plains." The Denver Post. May 12, 2011. https://www.denverpost.com/2011/05/12/when-deadly-dirt-devastated-the-southern-plains.

32. Williford, James. "Children of the Dust. The Dirty Thirties as Witnessed by People Who Were Actually There." *Humanities* 33, no. 6. National Endowment for the Humanities. November/December 2012. https://www.neh.gov/humanities/2012/novemberdecember/feature/children-the-dust.

33. Gordon, *Deadly Dirt.*

34. Wu, Yi-Chi, Ching-Sung Chen, and Yu-Jiun Chan. "The Outbreak of COVID-19: An Overview." *Journal of the Chinese Medical Association* 83, no. 3 (March 2020): 217–220. doi: 10.1097/JCMA.0000000000000270.

35. American Journal of Managed Care Staff. "A Timeline of COVID-19 Developments in 2020." *American Journal of Managed Care* (January 1, 2021). https://www.ajmc.com/view/a-timeline-of-covid19-developments-in-2020.

36. Shumaker, Lisa and Daniel Wallis, Editor. "U.S. Saw Summer of Black Lives Matter Protests Demanding Change." Reuters. U.S. News. December 7, 2020. https://www.usnews.com/news/top-news/articles/2020-12-07/us-saw-summer-of-black-lives-matter-protests-demanding-change.

37. Kishi, Roudabeh, and Sam Jones. "Demonstrations and Political Violence in America: New Data for Summer 2020." Armed Conflict Location and Event Data Project (ACLED). September 3, 2020. https://acleddata.com/2020/09/03/demonstrations-political-violence-in-america-new-data-for-summer-2020/. *Chapter 6*

Chapter 7

Failure to Regress to the Mean

SHOCKS TO THE SYSTEM

Human beings have a limited capacity for chaos, and act in predictable ways as we move outside the center of our torus. When a crisis hits, or is anticipated, we predictably panic-buy toilet paper and pasta.

When crisis-footing lasts, we crowd-in, as a means of self-soothing. We buy dogs, or bigger homes in the outer-ring suburbs, or build luxury patios, to bring an element of choice to a New Normal we did not choose for ourselves.[1]

The tactics we select to navigate this world will vary based on circumstance. But the mental flexibility needed for tough times, as well as the human susceptibility to finite voltage, is universal. We all have plenty to learn from each other. But no amount of learning exempts anyone from the risks we all face.

EMOTIONAL SUPPORT PEACOCK

In January 2018, a woman flying out of Newark, New Jersey made international news when she brought along an emotional support peacock for the ride.[2] An emotional support animal, in and of itself, is not controversial. They are not especially common, but every few times you flew, you might see a fellow flier, often a military veteran with a well-marked dog, with one. It was no big deal.

But with the emotional support peacock, it became clear that the emotional support trend had jumped the shark. Yesterday, your aisle-mate was an American with Disabilities Act (ADA) compliant service dog individually trained to do work or perform tasks for a person with a disability. Today, a peacock. Tomorrow, maybe, a baby bear?

This development was a slippery slope and we were traveling down it at warp speed. The integrity of the disability rights movement was also eroding as more and more pets were deemed "essential" by their owners.

The news was not just the oddity of the animal chosen for emotional support, though that was odd. Peacocks are not typically known for their companionship. No, the news was that someone finally said no. Enough was enough. United Airlines said the peacock was not welcome to fly the friendly skies.

Asked for its side of the story, United held firm. It said the peacock "did not meet guidelines for a number of reasons, including its weight and size," and that the woman had been told so three times before showing up at the airport with the bird anyway.[3]

Delta Airlines also spoke up and said that extreme comfort companions were a "disservice" to people with legitimate emotional needs.[4] "Customers have attempted to fly with comfort turkeys, gliding possums known as sugar gliders, snakes, spiders and more," Delta said in the statement. "Ignoring the true intent of existing rules governing the transport of service and support animals can be a disservice to customers who have real and documented needs."[5]

Two years after the peacock kerfuffle, emotional support animals (ESAs) lost their "protected" status on commercial American airlines altogether. According to the ESA Registration of America, a registry where people sign up their emotional support animals,

> As of January 2020, Emotional Support Animals are no longer considered a protected class of animal by US airlines. Airlines may now disallow ESA's on commercial flights or require travelers to pay a fee. Airlines that do allow ESA's require an ESA prescription letter from a licensed mental health professional as well as advance notice in most cases that the passenger will be flying with an ESA.[6]

Even if you sympathized with the emotionally in-need, you probably cheered the moves by United Airlines and Delta, and were happy to see the emotional support trend on the retreat.

Christmas Just Ain't Christmas If Every Day Is Christmas

The story of the emotional support peacock and its owner is what the news business calls a talker. It is the kind of story you forward to Mom or to your kids and enjoy a laugh at the ridiculousness of our times, always with a silent sigh.

You might be a picky eater or high maintenance, but you do not take it *that* far. It was all fun to watch from afar. Then the pandemic hit, and our own emotional support needs were laid bare.

Question: When did you take down your emotional support tree? Oh, sure, it was a Christmas tree when you got it. The snowfall and the smell of pine needles brought comfort in their own way. It has the feel and smell of nostalgia.

"When something that is physically or mentally encountered cues memory retrieval, we sometimes experience a distinct emotional state called nostalgia . . . nostalgia is now thought to serve a psychologically-adaptive function," reported a 2015 paper on the neuroscience of nostalgia.[7]

In 2018, the *Journal of Alzheimer's Disease* even found that "nostalgia helps enhance psychological resources—including social connectedness, meaning in life, self-continuity, optimism, self-esteem and positive mood— among people who have dementia."[8]

On our torus, we have spent months and months on the outer edge. The Christmas season, and its accoutrements, is the briefest of returns to the center. It takes the holiday of holidays to bring a sense of normalcy. Nostalgia can even help someone suffering dementia find their way back to the center.

In a pandemic-stricken year, tree shopping was a nice taste of the before-times. Even if the tree was fake. You knew and accepted that Christmas 2020 was going to be unlike any other. Maybe that trip over the river and through the woods to grandmother's house would not, or could not, happen this year. Perhaps, out of an abundance of caution, you would not see your nieces and nephews.

But there would be Christmas, and there would be a tree. You might not be at a big round table with everyone you love, but Christmas would be in your heart. A tree would stand in your living room. Then, one day, you woke up and the snow had melted and the smell of the pine needles faded and the twelve days of Christmas had passed.

There is always a little bit of a lag in getting the Christmas tree down. But a lag is not quite what happened this time. To call it a lag is to imply that taking the tree down is the ultimate plan. For so many people in 2021, keeping the tree up seemed the better move. At least at first. "We still have our Christmas tree up. And we're not alone. Do you have a problem with that, Chicago?" read the headline of a Valentine's 2021 story in *The Chicago Tribune*.[9]

The Christmas tree, a marker of winter, was transformed into a comfort item for all seasons, a celebratory item as fitting on Easter as the Fourth of July as Labor Day. This lack of distinction is akin to the difference between liking peacocks and deciding you cannot possibly get through a three-hour flight without one.

"My Christmas tree is still standing, and yes, it's artificial, but no, our household has made no movements toward taking it down," Christopher Borrelli confessed in *The Tribune*.[10] The Borrellis got an early start on things, hanging lights for Thanksgiving. By Valentine's Day the lights were approaching their fourth month in place. And they were not alone; Borrelli discovered when he spoke with his Chicagoland neighbors.

"It's rare to drive through a Chicago neighborhood or suburb right now without spotting a surprising number of February Christmas trees in our front windows," Borrelli wrote.[11] "There's even stray inflatable Christmas Minions on front lawns."[12]

In its original old English usage, holiday meant *holy day*. These were special days, often of religious significance. These were days off of work. Nowadays, the word *holiday* is more interchangeable with the word *vacation*, especially in Europe.

However the time is spent, what makes holidays special and set-apart from normal days are the rituals, the celebrations, and the freedom from obligation. In America, to the extent certain holidays are not also a day off, they are paid at time-and-a-half. These are special days indeed.

When red-letter days happen too often, they are just days. To stretch an already lengthy Christmas season across an entire calendar is the behavior of traumatized people. No one identifies themselves that way, and certainly not at the time. No one sets out to leave their Christmas tree up for a year. That happens one day at a time.

"It's not hard to assume why so many trees remain standing." Borrelli wrote.[13] "The pandemic, the economy, the state of American democracy, the gloom of a Chicago winter. Energy once spent repacking your lights is being expended on worrying."[14]

Crowd-in behavior not only meant that people were decorating for Christmas earlier and more robustly in 2020, but they were also reluctant to sunset the celebration by the Twelfth Night after Christmas (which was already confusing as people were mixed on the opinion of whether that was the 5th or 6th of January). According to lore, leaving a Christmas tree up after Twelfth Night means bad luck for the rest of the year.

An article in Great Britain's *The Guardian* stated that "English Heritage and Church of England back extending the traditional January deadline to brighten gloom of lockdown."[15]

Then, by seemingly divine intervention, *The Tablet—International Catholic News Weekly* fell in line and broke from the tradition of Epiphanytide, the culmination of the feast of Christmas and dropping the Christmas tree, and endorsed an extension on Christmas.[16]

Maybe you do not need a peacock, but after 2020, it is likely you will never again mock the idea of emotional support.

VOCABULARY TO LEXICON: 2020 CHANGED THE
DICTIONARY AND THE NEWS LIKE NEVER BEFORE

Never before had a dictionary entry changed so quickly.

Prior to October 2020, the phrase "sexual preference" was not widely, or even narrowly, considered offensive. It was understood to mean a person's dating preference. Nothing more, nothing less; that is, until the U.S. Senate confirmation hearings for the then-prospective Supreme Court Justice Amy Coney Barrett.

Senator Dianne Feinstein, D-California, asked if Barrett, a conservative jurist, would affirm gay marriage. Barrett answered that she had "never discriminated on the basis of sexual preference and would not ever discriminate on the basis of sexual preference."[17]

Mazie Hirono, a Democratic senator from Hawaii, challenged Barrett on that phrasing. "It is used by anti-LGBTQ activists to suggest that sexual orientation is a choice. It is not. Sexual orientation is a key part of a person's identity," Hirono said.[18]

She added: "If it is your view that sexual orientation is merely a preference . . . then the LGBTQ community should be rightly concerned whether you would uphold their constitutional right to marry."[19]

This was on a Tuesday. By Wednesday, *Merriam-Webster* had changed the dictionary entry for "preference" to note its use in the context of a "sexual preference" is "widely considered offensive."[20]

The change was not coincidental; it was caused directly by the discussion in the Senate hearing, and the rush to dictionary websites it inspired. *Merriam-Webster* admitted as much. *Merriam-Webster* explained that change is the nature of the business. If it were not, there would not be new editions printed each year. But the speed of the change, the character of the change, and the reason for the change were all unprecedented.[21]

The velocity of language was so powerful in 2020 that even the *dictionary* changed overnight. Dictionary definitions were driven by the twenty-four-hour news cycle, just like anything else. "From time to time, we release one or some of these scheduled changes early when a word or set of words is getting extra attention, and it would seem timely to share that update," *Merriam-Webster* editor-at-large Peter Sokolowski said in a statement to Fox News.[22]

"In this case, we released the update for sexual preference when we noticed that the entries for preference and sexual preference were being consulted in connection with the [Supreme Court] hearings," the statement continued.[23] People trust the dictionary to give accurate definitions.

But if this were a soccer match, *Merriam-Webster*'s actions would be the equivalent of a referee taking off their striped jersey and handing it to the parent yelling the loudest. No great shift in public opinion occurred overnight into Wednesday to make the phrase "sexual preference" "widely offensive," where it was not considered offensive at all on Monday.

In the end, Barrett apologized for her use of the now-offensive term "sexual preference," and was confirmed to the Supreme Court, filling the seat of the late Ruth Bader Ginsburg.

The change, the claim, and the timing all indicated that the studied judgment of Noah Webster had been supplanted by the senator and a few pointed tweets. For harmony's sake, Webster's successors seem to have decided that words mean whatever the most strident voices say they mean.[24]

Vocabulary and Lexicon, Protests and Pandemic

Between the COVID-19 pandemic, nationwide police brutality protests after the death of George Floyd, and the ever-expanding tentacles of political correctness, the events of 2020 added to our vocabulary and our lexicon at a speed never before seen.

Your vocabulary is the words you know. But increasingly, in 2020, those words became euphemisms.

Consider the "peaceful protest." A CNN chyron in August 2020, during a protest in Kenosha, Wisconsin, described the action as "fiery but mostly peaceful."[25] The video accompanying this description showed a violent riot with buildings actively on fire. CNN's claims were thus in direct conflict with what its own cameras showed the world. Who can you trust, when the Most Trusted Name in News is no longer in the truth business?

That term, "peaceful protest," was stretched yet again when then-president Donald Trump rebranded his in-person campaign rallies as "peaceful protests" that were then ostensibly First Amendment-protected exemptions from the stay-at-home orders across America. "If you can join tens of thousands of people protesting in the streets, gamble in a casino, or burn down small businesses in riots, you can gather peacefully under the 1st Amendment to hear from the President of the United States," the Trump campaign said at the time.[26]

In January 2020, a peaceful protest might have conjured an image of the Hash Bash in Ann Arbor, an annual combination music festival and civil disobedience event focused on reforming marijuana laws. By June 2020, the media calling violent riots a "peaceful protest" muddied the meaning. The words could no longer be trusted. Pictures, and consulting a multitude of sources, told the only real truth.

By October 2020, a "peaceful protest" could have meant anything from a kumbaya circle that cut off traffic on a main road, the torching of a downtown block, or a presidential campaign rally. Rarely have words been less instructive as to what had happened. You could only trust what you had seen with your own eyes.

The COVID-19 pandemic contributed not just to our vocabulary but it came with a lexicon all its own. Lexicon goes beyond vocabulary. With the words in your lexicon, the context is inherent and embedded in the meaning. People develop the lexicon of their career field. The pandemic was that rare circumstance when 300 million Americans all developed a shared lexicon at once. We were all in the same boat.

Consider the phrases "social distancing" and "contactless delivery." At the grocery store, if the person behind you in line is standing too close, simply saying the words "social distance" conveys not just information, but instruction. It reminds them, kindly, to move away.

The foundation for this new lexicon term was laid by countless press conferences and public service announcements. By that point in the store, it needs only to be invoked, not explained.

Because the expectations of "social distancing" were so well-established, alleged violations often escalated quickly. In August 2020, at a Colorado Springs Walmart, a sixty-year-old woman went from invoking social distancing to pushing the cart of the woman behind her to throwing that woman's items off the conveyor belt, according to a local TV news account.[27] The aggressor was not even wearing a mask at the time of a fight about social distancing, eyewitnesses told the news.[28]

Contactless delivery was another new lexicon word that tweaked the way we receive food, groceries, and packages. In a socially distant world, contactless options allowed people to stay home and have others do their shopping for them. Humans were still part of the process, and must then get the items to Point B. But those items were now left on the doorstep, rather than handed directly to the recipient.

Contactless delivery was as much a social contract as it was a New Normal. Timing is of the essence, and not just in the arrival of the food. Consider the pizza delivery driver that marks the delivery as complete while sitting in their car, and only then walks to the customer's front porch. The customer opens the door just as the delivery guy is leaving the pizza. That constitutes *contact*, exactly what the customer wanted to avoid, and the business promised she could by checking the appropriate box. A simple movement of the thumbs broke the promise of a contactless delivery.

The customer would have prepaid the tip by that point. The breach would bring no loss in the moment. But would that customer order from that pizzeria again? More likely, they would simply seek out a business that speaks their language and shares their lexicon.

REMOTE EVERYTHING—WE WERE
GOING TO GET HERE ANYWAY

After the COVID-19 pandemic hit, and after criminal courts in America returned on Zoom screens, rather than the courthouse, it opened the door for one of the most wasteful vestiges of the legal system to move online forever-more. Or at least begin in that direction.

Consider the calendar conference. In the before-times, a defendant in a criminal case had to take a day off of work, dress up, drive downtown, pay to park, and pay their attorney—all for a five-minute calendar conference, which usually just scheduled the next conference.

This process was inefficient and made the price of justice high for those caught in the court system. Every court date meant out-of-pocket expense and lost wages, at a minimum. But it was also the way things were done since time immemorial. Nowhere does precedent and inertia reign like in the court system. If the wheels of justice grind slowly, they do so proudly, and by design.

Maybe, the arc of justice would have eventually bent toward a more humane system for routine scheduling hearings. Perhaps someday, a pilot program to hold calendar conferences via Zoom would have been tried some-where, and worked, and been copied and become the standard. COVID-19 sped that timeframe up by at least a decade, bringing courts just warming to the technology of 2010 all the way into the world of 2030.

Sudden change is all but verboten in the court system until it becomes nec-essary. During the pandemic, the velocity of necessity changed the American court system by proving that scheduling matters can be handled via Zoom.

That change will far outlast the pandemic. There is no reason to go back to the charades of the past. Not when there are more considerate, even humane alternatives. Change usually requires a human catalyst. A champion. During the COVID-19 pandemic, necessity itself was that catalyst.

Zoom, of course, is not the best medium for *every* type of court date. Some things just need to be done in person.

In Detroit, in May 2021, a man was sentenced to up to fifteen years in prison in a domestic violence case.[29] The sentencing was held on Zoom, and Wayne County Circuit Judge Tracy Green gave the sentenced man, Adrian Brown, a day to report to Wayne County Jail.

This situation was a rare intersection of the justice system and the honor system, especially in a case involving violence. Had the sentencing been held in a courtroom, deputies would have taken the sentenced man into custody immediately and he would thereafter be transported to the prison system.

Giving the man a day to report really gave him a day to escape. Rather than report to jail as ordered, Brown cut his tether, allegedly kidnapped a woman in the suburbs, and led police in Southeast Michigan on a weeks-long manhunt.[30] The same technology that facilitated a safe court hearing had also opened the door to an escape, a kidnapping, and a manhunt.

The future was not ready for someone like Adrian Brown, but this also was not a failure of technology. This instance was a matter of human judgment. Zoom hearings work well for scheduling conferences but less so for sentencing hearings.

Zoom court hearings do not change the likelihood of adjournments and reschedulings—only their cost. By lowering it. A fifteen-minute scheduling conference can now happen during a defendant's lunch break, rather than costing him a day of work or the job itself.

Courts were going to get to that place eventually. Someday. Necessity just sped up the time frame. Avoiding change is impossible. Avoiding the consequences of change? Sometimes, that *is* possible.

JUST DO IT: COMPLIANCE BEHAVIOR TO AVOID CONSEQUENCES

Remember, in the early months of the pandemic, when you would get halfway through the grocery store parking lot, only to realize you had forgotten your mask? (figure 7.1) We have all been that person, patting our pockets, not feeling the mask, forced to turn back on that long march back to the car. Doing your part was not just worth the trip, it was your only way to get groceries. You did not love it, but you did it.

By early 2021, people had forgotten their masks too many times to forget them anymore. More than a year in, people were long past the early months' shouting matches with store security or other shoppers. It was not just easier to comply, it had become muscle memory.

So, you complied. You remembered the mask now. But maybe you waited until you were a foot outside the store to slip it on. Or maybe you pulled it off the second you set foot outside the store.

This game of chicken was not played with store clerks or security, but with yourself. It was a silent protest whose message to anyone watching is that you will be a good sport, you will do what is required; but nothing more, and not for a second longer than necessary. You have checked the box.

When was the last time you cleaned that mask, though, or switched it out? Its tattered condition made a statement of its own: that you could be ordered to mask up, but no one could make you care.

From day one, there was face validity incongruence between the messaging of the importance of wearing masks and generally accepted PPE protocols.

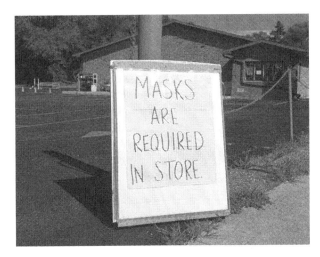

Figure 7.1   Masks Required Sign Outside of Wisconsin Thrift Store. *Credit David P. Perrodin.*

Imagine the entrance of the grocery store you patronize. Visualize it as modified so the incoming shopper was required to step into a biohazard hut to gown-up, put on a face shield, slip on gloves, and wear a store-issued mask that met stringent filtration criteria. And, when that person exited the store, they would enter another hut to deposit their PPE into a secure disposal unit.

That did not happen. None of the member checks reported that procedure (or a comparable virus-foiling stratagem) during their shopping experiences or when going to the post office to send a care package to grandma.

And then arrived the normalization of the mask as a fashion accessory. Global e-commerce site Etsy, an online marketplace for independent crafters, returned 1,238,558 results for the search query "Face Mask."[31] To Etsy's credit, the site clearly noted that items sold by its sellers, such as masks, are not medical grade and that Etsy sellers cannot make medical or health claims.

Others sought glitzy face coverings riveted with jewels (never mind the consequence of punching 100 holes in the life-saving fabric, right?) The effectiveness of the mask was secondary to its aesthetic swag—and that was fine with everyone. Store clerks were not dogging customers about the quality of their masks. In fact, they might be complimenting them for the nifty arrangement of white rhinestones on cloth.

Compliance behavior is that of the new hire who watches the sexual harassment seminar online, but on low volume; or the Catholic school student who attends Mass, but not in his heart. Compliance behavior is going through the motions.

Look up compliance behavior in a dictionary and you are likely to see a picture of former Seattle Seahawks running back Marshawn Lynch. Lynch was notoriously media-shy, but Super Bowl XLIX against the New England Patriots was a big enough deal, with big enough fines—$500,000 if he did not make himself available—that he was willing to break his silence. The NFL had made Lynch an offer he could not refuse.[32]

Held the week of the NFL Super Bowl, Media Day grants reporters the world over access to all of the players and coaches participating. Media Day is when the German TV network can get a few words with the offensive lineman *aus Deutschland*. Perhaps there are only five reporters at his booth, so those reporters each get more questions. It is the media's last chance to get everybody's last word.

Star players, like Lynch, draw a big crowd. His media hesitancy only made him more of a draw due to the rarity of the opportunity. The NFL had, finally, made him comply. But as reporters peppered Lynch with a season's worth of questions, he responded only by saying: "I'm just here so I don't get fined."[33]

"Y'all can sit here and ask me all the questions y'all want to," Lynch said in his opening remarks. "I'm gonna answer with the same answer."[34] Lynch's punchline turned into a headline. That headline traveled the world. By the year end Lynch had trademarked the phrase, and he even used it in a commercial for his favorite candy, Skittles.

Lynch was a Nike-sponsored athlete. Nike's slogan: Just Do It. Just Do It says nothing about liking it, whatever *it* may be. It is not the thought that counts, but the behavior. At Super Bowl Media Day, Lynch just did it. "I'm just here so I don't get fined" was not what reporters had asked for, or wanted. But it was something they could work with. By the end of Media Day, he had said "I'm just here so I don't get fined" *twenty-nine* times.[35]

The Seahawks lost the game, 28–24.

The Hawks were marching down the field. With about a minute left, Lynch was tackled on the 1-yard line. With everybody in the stadium and 100 million home viewers all thinking Lynch would be given the carry and score the touchdown giving the Seahawks the lead, Quarterback Russell Wilson instead threw a pass. Patriots' cornerback Malcolm Butler intercepted it at the goal line. Compliance with the coach's play call does not necessarily bring in championships, but nobody was cut, either.

Compliance Theater

Contrasted with the merely compliant are those who used the tools of fighting the pandemic—staying home and staying safe, social distancing, masks, and the vaccine—not only to ward off the virus but to build social cachet. Theirs was a performance of Compliance Theater. Among its prominent players was

President Joe Biden who regularly appeared masked and even double-masked months after being vaccinated.[36]

In March 2020, the participants in this security theater were staying home and urging that you should, too. This behavior assumed all Americans were subject to the same risk profile by the virus. By April 2020, our social media timelines were filled with posts such as, "Met a friend for a socially distanced walk."

At any point in the past, such a walk would have required an accompanying selfie of the participants. But this was a pandemic. If the lack of a selfie were not proof enough that your friend was taking this seriously, the accompanying hashtag left no doubt: #TakeThisSeriously.

By June 2020, they were confronting the unmasked in stores. Their social media posts wondered, aloud, why "caring about other people" was so hard to do. People liked those posts and said they, too, cared about other people.

When the vaccine came out, they predicated meetings with friends and even family on all parties being fully vaccinated. Mere compliance was not enough. Some people got "I'm vaccinated" tattoos. They had to be *seen* complying. They had to be *heard* complying. They had to be thought of by others as compliant. And they had to insist on your compliance, too. And if you would not do it for your own sake, then do it for the sake of others. Still not motivated? Here's a Krispy Kreme doughnut![37]

Compliance Theater during the COVID-19 pandemic was a game people played for marijuana edibles from the Mint Dispensary in Phoenix or doughnuts from Krispy Kreme.[38] Show your vaccination card for a cause and get a cure for the munchies.

Why did the government have to cajole people to accept a vaccine during a pandemic (when face validity would expect to observe people begging for it)? It is an upside down narrative. In California, the first two million residents to "start and complete their COVID-19 vaccination" received $50 gift cards.[39]

New Mexico went full *The Price is Right* and rolled out an impressive prize showcase. Its "Vax 2 the Max" sweepstakes included ten million dollars in winnings, free travel packages, fishing licenses, state park passes, and other prizes available to residents getting COVID-19 shots.[40] But that approach did not work in other places.

Folks were pouring through the exits in The Tar Heel State. North Carolina's million-dollar vaccine lottery, introduced on June 10, 2021, notched a weekly jab count of 115,000 vaccines—compared to 137,000 doses administered the week of May 31, 2021.[41]

People knew they could win one million dollars, with much better odds than Powerball, and the numbers showed they did not care. The attractions on stage no longer intrigued them. In response to the dismal data, Dr. David

Priest, an infectious disease specialist with Novant Health in Winston-Salem, said, "I think we reached a place where the individuals that are really interested in the vaccine have gotten that vaccine."[42]

When the novelty incentives go stale, people will stop participating because of the prizes. We will know we are officially past the pandemic when the curtain falls.

And what happens next? Nobody knows how this is likely to play out. What if doughnuts and sweepstakes are relics of halcyon days when all of us believed that we had a choice?

On July 12, 2021, French president Emmanuel Macron announced that France will make COVID-19 vaccination mandatory for health workers.[43] The compulsory measure is both about stomping out the stalwart strain of COVID-19 and walling off future variants. But as a prophylactic decree, it is also not transitory.

Proof of vaccination is increasingly required around the world for entry into restaurants, stadiums, universities, and for medical providers, transportation workers, and teachers.

We demanded information to arrive effortlessly by a mere tap and swipe. Now the velocity of information has reversed. Our personal information, from vaccination status to location, electronically radiates to our employers and the government through contact tracing apps downloaded onto our phones, including the places we do in-person commerce and our entertainment destinations.[44] It is no longer just informative, either. It is our passport to people, services, and experiences. Are you vaccinated? Are you essential?

TAKING OUR LIVES BACK

Nearly fifteen months to the day after the COVID-19 pandemic began, on May 13, 2021, the CDC announced that vaccinated people no longer needed to wear masks indoors or out.[45] Since the vaccinated and the unvaccinated cannot be told apart by looking, this announcement marked the end of the mask era. Because masks were the most visible sign of the pandemic, their removal marked its symbolic end.

Overnight, we went from socially distant, and even socially skeptical, to in-person, unmasked, and shaking hands like it was 2019. And this sudden snapback was not expected, right? Futurist Faith Popcorn prepared us for a lasting cocooned humanity. A great *retreat*, of sorts. It is simply a matter of time, according to Popcorn, before we live in pods and are brain-linked to the Internet, living a hologram life.

As we have fewer material needs, will we only become more neurotic? We are well far down that path now. We are stuck in our heads and have been discouraged from taking action. We look but do not touch. Subscribe or rent but do not own. And the kids growing up now are even more timid.

What would the equal and opposite reaction look like? Homesteading and homeschooling may resonate as ideas, in part due to that equal and opposite reaction. He who would build a perfect world must start small—perhaps in that cocoon.

Cocooning behavior is, and will remain, a transitory response to chaos events. It is not intended to be permanent, and never without an opt-out option. The cocoon is symbolic of living in a world of fear propped up by the quasi-religion of safe-ism.

Virtual wilderness hikes and hologram attendance at sporting events and concerts might be options from an array that includes the authentic experiences—one where you might step in gum. For those with circumstances that impede physical access, such as individuals with physical disabilities, alternatives, such as virtual reality hikes, will mean that the future is *more* inclusive than the present.

And, each person will be an arbiter of information. This book will always be relevant. There is no planned obsolescence for humans making the decisions to shape their lives and their world(s).

CHOOSE YOUR OWN HEALTH ADVENTURE

It used to be completely normal to pick up hitchhikers in America. It was never safe. But at one point it was normal.

And until about midway through 2020, it was not normal, in America, to wear a mask in public. In the early part of the year, when the pandemic was just a whisper, people would be called out in public for wearing masks and accused of stoking a climate of fear.

That tide quickly turned, and before long it was the mask-wearer who held the moral high ground. However, within a week of the May 13, 2021, CDC announcement, most grocery store chains in America matched the new federal guidance on masks.

But the masks did not go away immediately. For some they never will. Without fear of legal or social repercussions for going unmasked, and despite no social cachet to be had for masking up, some people still continue wearing them.

Why? Why not? They are doing what everybody should have done when the pandemic first hit: making a personal assessment of their health risks, and acting accordingly. Some people's health journeys take them to the gym or hiking trail. Others take them to the produce aisle, away from the processed food in the middle of the grocery store. For others still, down the mask aisle.

At its core, that is what *Velocity of Information* is all about: how to make the right decisions for yourself, and the people you love, in this chaotic, fast-changing world. Not what to do, which changes as the variables change, but how to curate your own attention and be liberated to think about it.

NOTES

1. Heller, Karen. "The New American Status Symbol: A Backyard That's Basically a Fancy Living Room." The Washington Post. May 25, 2021. https://www.washingtonpost.com/lifestyle/style/outdoor-furniture-patio-design-rug/2021/05/25/9199c7cc-b42b-11eb-9059-d8176b9e3798_story.html.

2. Silva, Daniella. "Emotional Support Peacock Denied Flight by United Airlines." NBC News. January 30, 2018. https://www.nbcnews.com/storyline/airplane-mode/emotional-support-peacock-denied-flight-united-airlines-n842971.

3. Silva, *Emotional Support Peacock.*

4. Delta Airlines. "Delta Introduces Enhanced Requirements for Customers Traveling with Service or Support Animals Effective March 1." Delta Airlines. June 4, 2020. https://news.delta.com/delta-introduces-enhanced-requirements-customers-traveling-service-or-support-animals-effective.

5. Delta Airlines, *Delta Introduces Enhanced Requirements.*

6. The Emotional Support Registration of America. "FAQs: Is an Emotional Support Animal (ESA) Allowed on a Plane?" ESA. (n.d.) https://www.esaregistration.org/faq/#:~:text=to%20top...-,Is%20an%20Emotional%20Support%20Animal%20(ESA)%20allowed%20on%20a%20plane,travelers%20to%20pay%20a%20fee.

7. Oba, Kentaro, Madoka Noriuchi, Tomoaki Atomi, Yoshiya Moriguchi, and Yoshiaki Kikuchi. "Memory and Reward Systems Coproduce 'Nostalgic' Experiences in the Brain." *Social Cognitive and Affective Neuroscience* (2016): 1069–1077.

8. Colino, Stacey. "How Nostalgia Can Be Good for Your Health and Well-Being." U.S. News & World Report. December 26, 2018. https://health.usnews.com/wellness/mind/articles/2018-12-26/how-nostalgia-can-be-good-for-your-health-and-well-being.

9. Borrelli, Christopher. "We Still Have Our Christmas Tree Up. And We're Not Alone. Do You Have a Problem With That, Chicago?" Chicago Tribune. February 14, 2021. https://www.chicagotribune.com/entertainment/ct-ent-christmas-lights-still-up-20210214-6dyftct5mnevraweee4dbyu4ui-story.html.

10. Borrelli, *We Still Have Our Christmas Tree Up.*

11. Ibid.

12. Ibid.

13. Ibid.

14. Ibid.

15. Bland, Archie and Alex Mistlin. "Light Brigade: The Christmas Holdouts Keeping Their Decorations Up." The Guardian. January 6, 2021. https://www.theguardian.com/uk-news/2021/jan/06/light-brigade-the-christmas-holdouts-keeping-their-decorations-up.

16. Carter, Michael. "Why It Is Time for an Epiphany Over Christmas Decorations." The Tablet—The International Catholic News Weekly. January 5, 2021. https://www.thetablet.co.uk/blogs/1/1682/why-it-is-time-for-an-epiphany-over-christmas-decorations.

17. Sopelsa, Brooke. "Amy Coney Barrett Apologizes for Use of Phrase 'Sexual Preference.'" NBC News. October 13, 2020. https://www.nbcnews.com/feature/nbc-out/amy-coney-barrett-apologizes-use-phrase-sexual-preference-n1243285.

18. Sopelsa, *Amy Coney Barrett Apologizes.*

19. Ibid.

20. Ibid.

21. Phillips, Morgan. "Merriam-Webster Changes Its Definition of 'Sexual Preference' as Barrett Gets Called Out for Using Term." Fox News. October 14, 2020. https://www.foxnews.com/politics/merriam-webster-changed-definition-sexual-preference-barrett-hearing.

22. Phillips, *Merriam-Webster Changes Its Definition of 'Sexual Preference.'*

23. Ibid.

24. Preference (October 14, 2020). In *Merriam-Webster's Collegiate Dictionary.* https://www.merriam-webster.com/dictionary/preference#usage-1.

25. Concha, Joe. "CNN Ridiculed for 'Fiery But Mostly Peaceful' Caption With Video of Burning Building in Kenosha." The Hill. August 27, 2020. https://thehill.com/homenews/media/513902-cnn-ridiculed-for-fiery-but-mostly-peaceful-caption-with-video-of-burning.

26. Colvin, Jill. "Trump Defies Virus Rules as 'Peaceful Protest' Rallies Grow." The Associated Press. September 20, 2020. https://apnews.com/article/donald-trump-election-2020-virus-outbreak-united-states-cff72c9f16ec77e3da073aca8c84e8de.

27. Dominguez, Alexis. "Fight Over Social Distancing at Colorado Springs Walmart Caught on Camera." KRDO-TV. August 3, 2020. https://krdo.com/news/2020/08/03/fight-over-social-distancing-at-colorado-springs-walmart-caught-on-camera/.

28. Dominguez, *Fight Over Social Distancing.*

29. Dickson, James. "Man Sought in Warren Kidnapping Was Sentenced to Prison Via Zoom Before Fleeing." The Detroit News. May 13, 2021. https://www.detroitnews.com/story/news/local/wayne-county/2021/05/13/warren-kidnapping-subway-zoom-prison-sentence-domestic-violence-fled/5059282001/.

30. Dickson, *Man Sought in Warren Kidnapping.*

31. Face Mask (product search query). Etsy. July 4, 2021. https://www.etsy.com/search?q=Face+Mask&ref=pagination.

32. Magary, Drew. "Holy Crap, The NFL Was Gonna Fine Marshawn Lynch $500K for Skipping Media Day." GQ. January 27, 2015. https://www.gq.com/story/holy-crap-the-nfl-was-gonna-fine-marshawn-lynch-500k-for-skipping-media-day.

33. Schilken, Chuck. "Watch Marshawn Lynch Answer All Media Day Questions the Same Way." Los Angeles Times. January 27, 2015. https://www.latimes.com/sports/sportsnow/la-sp-sn-marshawn-lynch-super-bowl-media-day-20150127-story.html.

34. Schilken, *Watch Marshawn Lynch.*

35. Ibid.

36. Hein, Alexandria. "Biden Got COVID-19 Vaccine and Still Wears 2 Masks: Doctors Weigh In." Fox News. March 10, 2021. https://www.foxnews.com/health/biden-covid-19-vaccine-2-masks.amp.

37. Tyko, Kelly and Robin Opsahl. "Krispy Kreme, Dunk' to Give Away Free Donuts Friday for Donut Day, Plus Get Extra with COVID Vaccine Card." Des Moines Register. June 3, 2021. https://www.desmoinesregister.com/story/enter-tainment/dining/2021/06/03/national-doughnut-donut-day-des-moines-iowa-dunkin-krispy-kreme-free-friday-deals-covid-vaccine-card/7527965002/.

38. deVaraona, Paola. "Here's All the Free Stuff You Can Get With Your COVID Vaccine Card." Verywell Health. April 12, 2021. https://www.verywellhealth.com/free-stuff-COVID-19-vaccine-5176144.

39. Kim, Soo. "Vaccine Lottery by State and How to Enter." Newsweek. June 4, 2021. https://www.newsweek.com/covid-vaccine-lottery-state-how-enter-1597502.

40. Grisham, Michelle Lujan. "New Mexico Launches 'Vax 2 the Max' Sweepstakes." Office of the Governor. State of New Mexico. June 1, 2021. https://www.governor.state.nm.us/2021/06/01/new-mexico-launches-vax-2-the-max-sweepstakes/.

41. Lundberg, Rachel. "VERIFY: No, the $1 Million Lottery Hasn't Led to More Vaccinations in North Carolina." WCNC-TV Charlotte. June 23, 2021. https://www.wcnc.com/article/news/verify/verify-north-carolina-vaccine-lottery-increase-vacci-nation-rate-data/275-581482ac-149e-454e-a216-f813ad7ce308.

42. Lundberg, *VERIFY: No, the $1 Million Lottery Hasn't Led to More Vaccinations.*

43. Gouvy, Constantin and Angela Charlton. "French Rush to Get Vaccinated After President's Warning." Associated Press. July 13, 2021. https://apnews.com/arti-cle/europe-business-lifestyle-health-travel-1d10271c4f1617521892d49d83b773ad.

44. Winder, Davey. "How to Disable Apple and Google's COVID-19 Notifications on Your Phone." Forbes. June 28, 2020. https://www.forbes.com/sites/daveywinder/2020/06/28/how-to-disable-apple-and-googles-covid-19-notifications-on-your-phone-coronavirus-tracking-and-contact-tracing-app/?sh=34175cbb7242.

45. Wamsley, Laurel. "Fully Vaccinated People Can Stop Wearing Masks Indoors and Outdoors, CDC Says." National Public Radio (NPR). May 13, 2021. https://www.npr.org/2021/05/13/996582891/fully-vaccinated-people-can-stop-wearing-masks-indoors-and-outdoors-cdc-says.

Epilogue
The Great Re-Greet

Remember those cute pandemic puppies adopted by the crate load as the quarantined looked to ameliorate their loneliness? As the pandemic restrictions were lifted, people perceived an end to uncertain times and discontinued their crowding-in behavior. People began leaving their homes and socializing again. The need for a furry companion to stave off loneliness decreased. And many of those dogs ended up back at the animal shelter.[1]

When I started out writing this book, my plan was to find the superhumans among us. I was going to identify, interview, and study those among us who handle change and bad circumstance with machine-like efficiency, and report back their tactics for the rest of us mere mortals to learn from their actions.

While there is plenty to learn, my very first lesson is that there are no superhumans. Superman does not appear in these pages. The people you have met are more like Clark Kent, the news reporter. Their superpowers do not come from changing clothes in the phone booth, but from working the phones.

Whether they were in prison, on a southern homestead, or in the U.S. Army Special Forces, the people you have met herein sought out and found truth by utilizing a variety of sources.

Velocity of Information is an assemblage of stories and characters, yes. But more than that, it is a study of mediums and messages and messengers. It draws from war and peace, from natural disasters and nuclear crises, from propaganda and pandemic.

All of the evidence still has to be weighed and measured. Human reason and human judgment will always matter. Before we even consult with other people, we evaluate claims on a face validity level.

If, on July 1, a friend told you it was snowing in Death Valley, California, you probably would not rush to go check CNN. The odds would seem roughly impossible.

On first impression, your friend's claim is more of a bad joke than a good prank. It is not compelling because it lacks face validity. Pranks like the above do not work anymore because there is no information gap these days.

In the 2020 movie *News of the World*, set five years after the end of the American Civil War, Tom Hanks played a newsman who went town to town reading the newspaper aloud for people who paid him.[2] Before there were newsreels, there were news readings, wherein a literate man with possession of a newspaper would share the news of the world with those lacking the time or need for a novel's worth of true stories.

News stories that inspire conversation are called "talkers." If you were not up on the news, what would you have to say when you visited town, or returned home from it? As stoic and dignified as we believe our ancestors to be, not even they were immune to fear of missing out.

More than a century ago, news was a strictly opt-in experience. People plunked down cash to read true stories, or to have those stories read to them, or to watch short news clips at the local theater.

Today, because of the smartphone we tether to our own hands, people can hardly opt out. Because we are never unplugged from the news, we have lost the ability to break news to one another. We are never out of the loop of the news, and so there is no need for us to be brought up to speed. Consequently, attention has been captured by our devices, and we have been robbed of the basic emotions of anticipation and surprise.

If there were record-setting snows falling in Death Valley, rest assured the push alerts on your phone or your Twitter timeline would have alerted you long before your friend's breathless announcement. When your indicators are not indicating anything, that is usually because there is nothing to indicate.

However, we have also learned that attention to indicators, and evaluating them properly through the methods described can also be of critical importance in both the initial stages of a crisis event and for the duration of an extended chaos event. Making decisions about the information collected can lead to several psychological responses, such as crowding-in behavior, as we try to maintain our torus.

My original title for the closing of this book was "It is going to be an interesting few days for the next ten years." I anticipated an incremental wind-down of uncertain times followed by drawn-out social guidance campaigns similar to the post–World War II Coronet Instructional Films that were shown in American schools; perhaps contemporary remakes of *Everyday Courtesy* (1948) or *The Benefits of Looking Ahead* (1950).[3]

I undervalued the human spirit's ability to re-animate itself. In support of my fell-short prediction, much of this book was written in vivo 2020.

People are capable of surviving incredible hardship and sacrifice when circumstances require it. But when that crisis ends, they want their lives back.

This desire is our preprogrammed need to return to our torus. And I wonder if such a return is even possible in this age of rapid information transfer. We are now not simply receiving information, but are sending it back out to the world, both voluntarily and involuntarily, at an ever-increasing rate.

Where will this *Velocity of Information* lead us in the future?

NOTES

1. Romaine, Jenna. "Pandemic Puppies Returned to Shelters as COVID-19 Restrictions Lift." The Hill, May 12, 2021. https://www.thehill.com/changing -america/sustainability/environment/553226-pandemic-puppies-returned-to-shelters -as-covid-19.

2. *News of the World.* Directed by Paul Greengrass. Universal Pictures, 2020. https://www.universalpictures.com/movies/news-of-the-world.

3. *Everyday Courtesy.* Coronet Instructional Films, 1948. Public Domain. https:// archive.org/details/Everyday1948 and *The Benefits of Looking Ahead.* Coronet Instructional Films, 1950. Public Domain. https://archive.org/details/Benefits1950.

Index

Note: Italic page numbers refer to figures.

About the Author

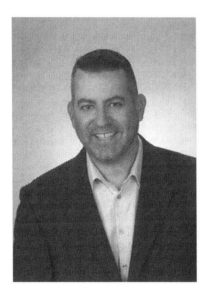

Figure A.1 **David P. Perrodin.** *Credit Fred Galley.*

David P. Perrodin, Ph.D., is the wrangler of nonlinear things that are impossible to predict or control. He is an author, researcher, professor, and host of *The Safety Doc Podcast*. Dr. Perrodin earned his Doctor of Philosophy degree in Educational Leadership and Policy Analysis from the University of Wisconsin-Madison where he researched high-stakes safety decisions in education, healthcare, and the military.

He has delivered two school safety presentations on Wisconsin Public Television that have been distributed through the Public Broadcasting System (PBS) network, and also wrote and directed a film about school safety with Pulitzer Prize winner David Obst.

Dr. Perrodin's work has been published in a number of journals and he is frequently interviewed by the media about school safety topics. He is the author of the book *School of Errors: Rethinking School Safety in America.*[1]

NOTE

1. Perrodin, David P. *School of Errors: Rethinking School Safety in America* (Lanham, MD: Rowman & Littlefield, 2019).

Made in the USA
Columbia, SC
26 March 2023

14335683R00126